The View From My Window

A Personal Account from an Eye Cancer Survivor

Cindy A. Nightingale

The View From My Window
Copyright © 2020 by Cindy A. Nightingale

All rights reserved. No part of this publication may be reproduced, distributed, or transmitted in any form or by any means, including photocopying, recording, or other electronic or mechanical methods, without the prior written permission of the author, except in the case of brief quotations embodied in critical reviews and certain other non-commercial uses permitted by copyright law.

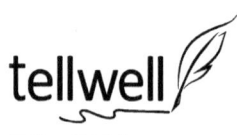

Tellwell Talent
www.tellwell.ca

ISBN
978-0-2288-4083-1 (Paperback)
978-0-2288-4751-9 (Hardcover)
978-0-2288-4084-8 (eBook)

DISCLAIMER

I Am Not A Doctor

All content found in *The View From My Window: A Personal Account From an Eye Cancer Survivor* or on the NightingaleCreations.ca website, including text, images, audio, or other formats were created for informational purposes only. The content is not intended to be a substitute for professional medical advice, diagnosis, or treatment. Always seek the advice of your physician or other qualified health provider with any questions you may have regarding a medical condition. Never disregard professional medical advice or delay seeking it because of something you have read in this story or on this website. *The View From My Window: A Personal Account From an Eye Cancer Survivor* or the NightingaleCreations.ca website does not recommend or endorse any specific tests, physicians, products, procedures, opinions, or other information that may be mentioned on NightingaleCreations.ca. Reliance on any information provided by *The View From My Window: A Personal Account From an Eye Cancer Survivor* or the NightingaleCreations.ca website is solely at your own risk.

Legal Disclaimer: All photographs displayed in this publication or on this website are the sole property of Cindy A. Nightingale, Nightingale Creations, *The View From My Window: A Personal Account From an Eye Cancer Survivor*. All other content in this publication or on this website is owned by Cindy A. Nightingale, Nightingale Creations, *The View From My Window: A Personal Account From an Eye Cancer Survivor*. Except as expressly authorized by Cindy A. Nightingale, Nightingale Creations, *The View From My Window: A Personal Account From an Eye Cancer Survivor* herein, you agree not to copy, modify, rent, lease, loan, sell, assign, distribute, license, reverse engineer, or create derivative works based on the website or any content available through the website.

*To my amazing husband and best friend,
Gary Nightingale. You stood by my side and were
my guiding light during the most difficult time of my life.
Thank you for your love, encouragement, and support.*

Photo Caution

Caution: *The View From My Window: A Personal Account From an Eye Cancer Survivor* contains some pictures that were taken immediately following eye removal surgery and may be disturbing to some. Due to the graphic nature of these pictures, viewer discretion is advised.

TABLE OF CONTENTS

Preface: A Note From the Author ix
Acknowledgements xi

Chapter 1.   Happy Tears 1
Chapter 2.   The First Sign of Trouble 5
Chapter 3.   The Discovery 8
Chapter 4.   Preparations and Reflections 12
Chapter 5.   Road Trip 17
Chapter 6.   Disturbing Diagnosis 21
Chapter 7.   Making Time for Metal 30
Chapter 8.   Our Graduate 34
Chapter 9.   The Waiting Period 37
Chapter 10. Back to Toronto 40
Chapter 11. Life-Altering Surgery 43
Chapter 12. Seeing Things Differently 55
Chapter 13. Healing at Home 57
Chapter 14. Looking Normal? 68
Chapter 15. Cancer Screening 81
Chapter 16. Wedding Bells 88
Chapter 17. New Eye Complications 93
Chapter 18. Dark Days 97
Chapter 19. Starting Over 100
Chapter 20. Walking in Her Footsteps 103

PREFACE: A NOTE FROM THE AUTHOR

On May 18, 2004, I was told I had a mass in my eye, specifically in my iris. At thirty-six years old, I was beyond shocked and terrified. I frantically searched the internet for information but found very little, and certainly nothing that prepared me for what was about to happen. I decided to track my experience through journal entries and photos in an effort to help others who were looking for information for themselves, a friend, or a family member. Unfortunately, I did not foresee how traumatizing my journey would be or how painful it would be to recount my experience. Over the years, I tried many times to complete this memoir but it was too painful and upsetting. Time and time again, I shelved it, all the while feeling guilty about not sharing my experience with those who came after me.

Due to debilitating inflammatory polyarthritis and fibromyalgia, I resigned from my position as a supervisor for a financial institution in 2015. This left me feeling frustrated, bored, and unsure about what I could do with my life that was productive and meaningful. My medical issues, tests, and appointments took up a fair bit of my time, but I still felt like I could be doing something useful on my good days. With the encouragement of my husband, Gary, I decided to finally finish my memoir. I was hesitant, as reading my journal entries usually made me extremely depressed, but I was determined to finish it this time.

ACKNOWLEDGEMENTS

To my son, Matt Nightingale: I sincerely thank you for your insight. Your vast knowledge of a great number of things has helped me immensely throughout this process. You have grown into a kind and considerate man and have become one of my closest friends.

Gratitude and thanks to my mother-in-law, Muriel Nightingale: having lived most of my life without my own mother, your gentle demeanour and kind heart has had a profound impact on my life.

To my best friend, Sherri Chenard: thank you for your lifelong friendship. Your sense of humour, compassion, and sense of adventure have added a great deal to my life.

To Jeff Chase, Jeff Chase Photography: thank you for being a wonderful friend and always being there when we needed you. You dropped everything at the last minute, came to our wedding, and took such beautiful photos. We will forever cherish them.

To Chuck Wilby: thank you for being a lifelong, loyal friend. You are a kind, generous man and would gladly give the shirt off your back to help someone in need.

To Dr. Hugh McGowan, BSc, MD, FRCS(C): thank you for saving my life. Words cannot possibly express my gratitude. You are a king among men. What would be an insurmountable task for most was just Thursday for you.

To the late Dr. John W. Purdy, BSc, MSc, PhD, MD: you also played a huge part in saving my life. You recognized the seriousness of my condition and took the necessary steps to keep me safe while I awaited surgery. You will be fondly remembered.

To Daphne Archibald, BCO, BADO, Archibald Maxillofacial Prosthetics Inc.: thank you for your expertise and your kindness. You were not the first ocularist to work on my prosthetic eye, but you were certainly my favourite by far. You taught me a great deal about prosthetic eyes, orbital implants, the process, and the complications. You worked your magic on many occasions and made me look and feel beautiful.

To Dr. Alejandra A. Valenzuela, MD: thank you for taking away my pain and giving me my life back. The impact you had on my life is immeasurable.

To the Princess Margaret Ocular Oncology Clinic and those who work there: thank you for your thorough testing, professionalism, and empathy. It did not go unnoticed.

To Dr. James McKim, MD, and Dr. Susan Dempsey, MD, my family physicians: thank you both for your kindness and your excellent, personalized care over the years.

To many other wonderful family members, awesome friends, and various medical professionals: you have all had a great impact on my life, and I will be forever grateful.

CHAPTER 1

HAPPY TEARS

I was packing when the phone rang. It was my boyfriend, Gary; he said he had hurt his back and needed me to come to the new house right away. It was July 1, 2003, the day Gary and I took possession of our house in Fredericton, New Brunswick. I was hopeful it wasn't anything serious. I immediately dropped everything, grabbed my keys, and headed toward the house.

By this point, Gary and I had already been together for several years. I knew he was the right person for me after our first conversation as he showed me a level of kindness and compassion I hadn't felt in a long time. He was also incredibly handsome, standing over six feet tall with dark hair, a muscular build, and a playful smile; I was immediately captivated. Gary had started an IT business from scratch and turned it into a thriving company, but his great love was music. When we met, he was a drummer in a progressive metal band that often played at local venues and had just released a CD. Eventually the band broke up, but Gary was not deterred and continued to play drums and guitar as well as write and record songs in his home studio.

Through the years, our love grew strong as we realized we had everything in common including a sarcastic sense of humour that we shared with my son, Matt. Gary had been in my son's life since he was seven years old. They had a close relationship and a number of common interests including video games and music. Matt was extremely intelligent, almost fluently bilingual and excelled in school, especially in math. He was kind and sensitive, made friends easily, and had a great love for animals. In the fall, he would be going into his final year of high school, but there was a complication: the new house was located in another school district twenty minutes away. Matt would either have to switch schools or be driven to and from his current school as he would be outside of the bus route. Gary and I decided to drive Matt so he could graduate with his lifelong friends. It would be a great deal of scheduling and driving, but it would be well worth the effort.

Turning onto our street, I admired the countless mature green and red maple trees lining the sidewalk providing shade on that hot summer day. I pulled into the driveway of our new house. It was an older bungalow that had been in Gary's family for decades. It had become too much for his aging mother to care for, so she sold it to us and moved into an apartment. Gary and I planned to renovate it over the next few years to transform it into the home of our dreams.

I walked into the house and called out to Gary; he yelled back saying he was in the master bedroom. My footsteps echoed as I ran through the empty house. I wondered how badly he was hurt and if I would need to take him to the hospital. When I reached the doorway, I expected to see him lying on the floor in agony but, to my surprise, Gary was down on one knee grinning from ear to ear. He was holding a tiny black box containing a beautiful diamond solitaire ring set in white gold. I was surprised and elated. I knew I wanted to marry Gary within our first few months together, but I wanted him to ask me when he was ready. Gary then said the four words I had been patiently waiting to hear: "Will you marry me?"

Tears filled my eyes as I said, "Yes, of course I'll marry you!"

Gary also said he wanted to complete our family by adopting Matt. Dancing around our empty master bedroom, I realized I was happier than I'd ever been in my life. I felt incredibly fortunate to be engaged to such an amazing man, and I was looking forward to the road ahead of us.

Our family included our two lovable, furry friends: Jody, our seven-year-old black Labrador retriever, and Kitty, our eight-year-old black cat. We fenced in the back yard of our new place for Jody, but we were a bit worried about Kitty since he was an outside cat in an unfamiliar neighbourhood. Three days after we moved in, Kitty went outside and didn't come back. We looked for him constantly, spending countless hours walking around our neighbourhood while calling for him, but he was nowhere to be found. We were all so sad as he was such an integral part of our household. He adored Matt and spent a lot of time with him, sleeping on his bed at night and sitting on his desk while he did his homework. Kitty and Jody were also very close and would often have naps together or take turns chasing each other around the yard.

Three weeks later, I drove out to our old place in Lincoln. I had been going back every couple of days to finish cleaning and painting as we were getting it ready to sell. As I drove into the driveway, Kitty came running towards the car meowing and meowing. Tears filled my eyes as I scooped up my sweet cat with his big yellow eyes, shiny black fur, and extra toes that made it look like he had thumbs. He had lost a few pounds and looked distraught but somehow, he had made it all the way from our new house back to our old house ten kilometers away. I immediately put him into the car and drove back home as I was sure he was starving. When we arrived at the new house, I brought Kitty in, gave him a can of food and called out to Gary to come into the kitchen. Gary was elated to see Kitty and Kitty was just as happy to see him. Gary pet him while he purred and ate and occasionally meowed. When Matt came home, Kitty ran to the door to greet him; Matt was so relived and excited to see him. He told me he had been holding out hope for Kitty and believed he was okay and would eventually come home. We bought a harness and a long leash to walk Kitty, hoping to familiarize him with our new neighbourhood. He was not happy about the leash and would often struggle to get out of his harness. After a few days, we all agreed to let him go free as he was so unhappy and would constantly cry; fortunately, it worked, and he never got lost again.

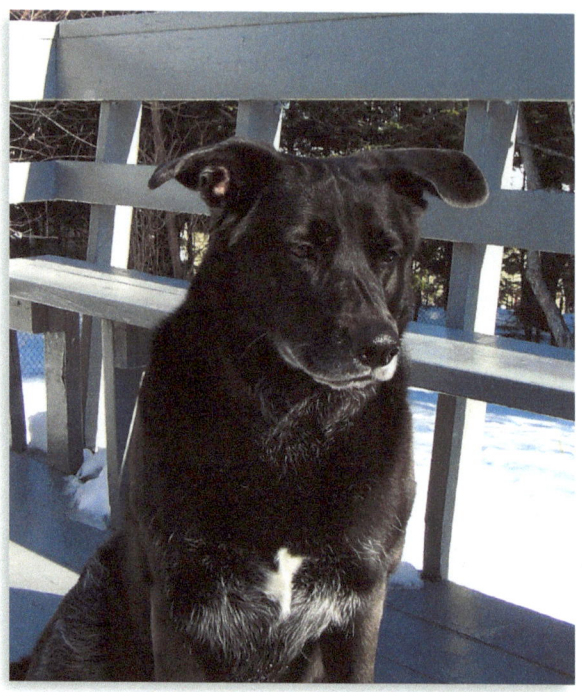

Jody, our seven-year-old black Labrador retriever.

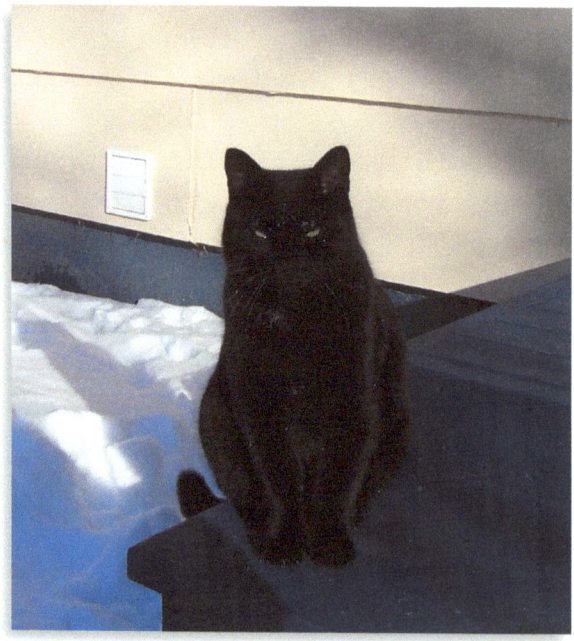

Kitty, our eight-year-old black cat.

CHAPTER 2

THE FIRST SIGN OF TROUBLE

The following year was a challenge to say the least. Gary and I were both working full time and sharing the responsibility of driving Matt to and from school each day. We struggled to carve out time to spend together especially since I had taken a later shift and was working most weekends. Each morning when my alarm went off, I felt more tired than the last. I had never been a morning person and having to get up early after working an evening shift was painful, especially since I knew I would be up for a few hours while driving my tired teenager to school. It made for some rough mornings. Gary was also feeling a little overwhelmed knowing he would have to stop working everyday by 3:30 p.m. so he could pick up Matt from school. As difficult as it was, Gary and I enjoyed our talks with Matt during our daily drives; he would tell us about his day and about his future plans and ambitions. It helped to know it was Matt's final year of high school.

One afternoon near the end of February, I was staring out our living room window when I called Gary at his office. I had stayed home from work due to a bad cold, but I had another problem I could no longer ignore. I realized every time I coughed or sneezed my right eye would cloud over for a few seconds. A month earlier I had noticed my eye was cloudy at times; I thought it was caused by my contact lenses. I stopped wearing them and the issue went away, but when I got sick the issue returned. I had been avoiding mentioning it to Gary because I didn't want to worry him, but it was getting worse and I couldn't put it off any longer. My heart pounded hard in my chest as I told him about my cloudy eye. Saying it out loud made it real. Until that point, I had been trying my best to ignore the issue, hoping it would go away on its own. Gary was concerned and recommended I make a doctor's appointment right away.

I immediately called my family doctor's office, but the receptionist told me they were booked solid and she wouldn't be able to fit me in for a couple of weeks. She recommended I visit an after-hours medical clinic or, if it was urgent, go to the hospital emergency room. I didn't want to wait any longer so that evening I went to an after-hours medical clinic with the hope the doctor would be able to alleviate my concerns.

Walking into the clinic, I wondered if being there was a mistake. It was crowded with at least thirty people, including several babies and young children. I wondered if I should've just made a doctor's appointment instead of taking up the clinic doctor's time with what was likely a simple eye infection.

After waiting for a few hours, I finally saw the doctor on duty. He was a tall, dark-haired man with a round, young face. He looked somewhat confused when I described my symptoms. The doctor covered my left eye and asked me to read some letters off an eye chart taped to the back of the examination room door. My vision was cloudy, as if I was trying to see through a dirty window, but I was still able to read the letters. He said the cold virus had likely moved into my eye, and if the issue didn't go away within a couple of weeks, I should make an appointment to see my family doctor. I left the clinic feeling skeptical of the diagnosis, especially since I didn't have any of the common symptoms associated with having a cold virus in my eye, such as swelling, itchiness, or discharge.

By the middle of March, the vision in my right eye was still occasionally cloudy but my cold was gone. As directed by the doctor from the medical clinic, I made an appointment with my family doctor. Two weeks later,

I explained my issue to my doctor and I was immediately referred to an ophthalmologist named Dr. Purdy. I already knew him as my son was his patient when he was just four years old. Matt had a condition called amblyopia (lazy eye), but with treatment his condition improved, and he hadn't required an ophthalmologist for the past decade.

A month later, I was feeling stressed as my eye issue was getting much worse and I still hadn't heard from Dr. Purdy's office. Instead of being cloudy for a few seconds or minutes at a time, my eye was often cloudy for a few hours at a time. I called Dr. Purdy's office directly and his receptionist told me it could take a few months to be scheduled for an appointment. I described my symptoms and pleaded with her to fit me in to see the ophthalmologist as soon as possible. She said Dr. Purdy was planning to add an extra day for urgent patients and she would call and let me know once it was added to his schedule. Less than a week later, to my great relief, the receptionist called with an appointment for the following week.

CHAPTER 3

THE DISCOVERY

Finally, it was May 18, 2004, the day of my ophthalmologist appointment. I was relieved someone with authority would be looking at my eye. I was frustrated with how long it had taken to get an appointment to see a specialist as I was concerned there was something seriously wrong. I did a little research and it seemed like I might have cataracts, glaucoma, or an infection.

I would normally take my own car but since I would be getting drops in my eyes to dilate my pupils, Gary drove me to my appointment. When we arrived at the medical centre, we took the elevator to the fourth floor, walked down a long hallway, and into Dr. Purdy's empty waiting room. Gary took a seat while I checked in with the receptionist. I was immediately taken into an examination room and after a couple of minutes, Dr. Purdy came in. He hadn't changed much since I had seen him last. He had a few more lines on his face and his grey hair had turned white, but he still had the same kind eyes and gentle demeanour. He put drops into both of my eyes and then ran a battery of tests.

When the tests were finished, Dr. Purdy asked me if I had experienced any type of head trauma—had I been hit in the head with a baseball or anything? I was surprised by his questions; they made me wonder what he saw in my eye. I said I hadn't.

"Can you go to Toronto?" he said.

It was the last thing I was expecting him to say and I didn't know how to answer him. I wasn't sure if Gary and I could afford to go. What about Matt, our pets, and my job? I'd have to discuss it with Gary. All I could muster as a response was, "Why?" Dr. Purdy had his back to me and was writing something in my chart. Without looking up, he calmly said, "You have a mass in your eye." His words echoed in my ears. I was in shock. Dr. Purdy told me the mass was creating an excessive amount of pressure, causing glaucoma and causing my retina to detach. This explained my cloudy vision. He went on to tell me about the specialists at the Ocular Oncology Clinic in the Princess Margaret Hospital in Toronto. At that point my fear reached its peak. I started panicking; nothing he was saying made sense. I had to find Gary and tell him what was happening.

As I walked hurriedly toward the waiting room, my mind was racing. I thought, *This can't be happening, I thought it was just an infection. A mass in my eye? Is that the same thing as a tumour? He wants me to go to Toronto. It must be serious; what if it's cancer? Can you even get cancer in your eye and, if so, how do they treat it? I can't believe I have to tell my fiancé this news, it's going to break his heart.* I rounded the corner to be faced with an empty waiting room; I was surprised and disappointed Gary had left. Then it hit me: I had been in the examination room for almost an hour and Gary had to pick up Matt from school. We had made the arrangement before my appointment, but it had completely slipped my mind. I was grateful Gary was picking up Matt but, at that moment, I felt terrified and alone.

I broke down sobbing uncontrollably. I ran out of the office and down the long hallway. I could hardly see through my tears, and I was sobbing so hard I could barely breathe. I ran into the washroom and looked at my red, puffy face in the mirror. I tried to persuade myself to calm down and call Gary. I took my phone out of my purse to dial his number, but I kept breaking down. I knew I needed to pull myself together, but I was afraid

I had just been handed a death sentence. I couldn't stop sobbing. I finally took a deep breath, composed myself, and called him. I could hardly get the word "mass" out before I started sobbing again. Hearing Gary's voice was comforting; he reassured me we would get through this together. He said we would definitely go to Toronto and get the best doctors available. I was grateful to have him on my side, but I knew all the love and support in the world couldn't protect me from cancer. Gary told me Matt was just getting into the car and they were going to come back to pick me up. We decided we would wait until we got home to tell Matt the news.

When I hung up the phone, I started to tear up again, but then a mother and her two young children came into the washroom; out of concern for the children, I pulled myself together and left. I walked back down the long hallway and into the ophthalmologist's office. I asked the receptionist about the Toronto hospital and who I needed to contact. Dr. Purdy must have heard my voice because he immediately came out of his office. He told me I would get a call from someone at the Princess Margaret Hospital who would give me an appointment for the Ocular Oncology Clinic. He then handed me a prescription for some drops and pills to bring down the pressure in my eye (Diamox 500MG Sequels and PMS Timolol 0.5% opts dr) and told me he was out of the office the following week, but he would have another ophthalmologist contact me to check my eye pressure to make sure the medication was working.

I left the office feeling numb. Again, I walked down the long hallway, this time stopping in front of the elevator. I pushed the down button and it turned red. As I stood there waiting, I was dumbfounded. I could not believe what was happening. I knew something was wrong with my eye, but I never imagined I'd be told I had a mass in it.

I was sixteen years old when my mother found a large lump in her breast. I could see the look of fear on her face when she told me about it. She tried to reassure me, telling me it might not be cancer, but I was worried. At my young age, I was familiar with the devastating power of cancer as one of my mother's best friends had recently died from breast cancer, and my paternal grandfather had lost his voice box to cancer a few years before. I waited and agonized for what felt like hours in a hospital waiting room while my mother had her biopsy. Finally, the doctor came in and said her lemon-sized breast tumour was cancer and it had spread to some of her lymph nodes. He was immediately taking her into surgery to remove her breast and the affected lymph nodes. I was devastated. The thought of losing my mother was terrifying as she was my anchor, my closest confidant, and I loved her dearly.

I desperately hoped I wasn't headed down the same path as my mother. I went down the elevator and walked outside for some fresh air. The sunny sky had clouded over, and the wind had picked up. I zipped up my jacket and sat down on the rough, cold concrete steps while I waited for Gary and Matt to arrive.

CHAPTER 4

PREPARATIONS AND REFLECTIONS

When we got home, Gary and I sat down with Matt and broke the news to him about the mass in my eye. We told him I had to go to Toronto to see some specialists who would determine exactly what it was and what needed to be done to get rid of it. He was very calm, which was his character, and asked a few questions about how long we would be gone and what I was told by the ophthalmologist. We told him everything we knew; he was concerned but optimistic. He immediately offered to take care of the pets and the house while we were gone. Gary and I were proud of our brave, considerate son and we greatly appreciated his offer to help during such a difficult time.

Over the next few days, Gary and I made quite a few phone calls to inform our family and friends about my situation and our upcoming trip to Toronto. Everyone was supportive and concerned and asked for regular updates. Anytime I looked worried, Gary would comfort me and tell me not to jump to any conclusions. He said I should look into things I wanted to do while we were in Toronto and think of our trip as a mini vacation. I tried to think positive, but I couldn't help searching the internet for any information I could find to help me understand what was about to happen to me. I found some medical journal entries describing various treatments for eye tumours and tried to decipher the medical language, but I was only able to understand bits and pieces. The least invasive treatment was something called plaque radiation therapy. In this treatment, a thin piece of metal was attached to the surface of the eye and would deliver a high dose of radiation to shrink the mass, but it was only for specific types of tumours. Most of the recommended treatments involved removal of the eye. As unbelievable as it was, I had to somehow come to terms with the fact that I was probably going to lose my eye.

My journal entry four days after I was told about the mass in my eye shows my frustration with the lack of progress.

> *Saturday, May 22, 2004*
>
> *I am horrified that no one has called yet from the doctor's office. I was supposed to see another eye specialist on Thursday or Friday to check the pressure in my eye and see if the medication is working. They just don't care! It's not their problem! And I'm still waiting for the call about Toronto and when I go! The doctor said they would call in a day or so with the info. I hate waiting! I don't even know how long I'll be there or where we'll stay. It is so irritating. I just want to get on with it.*

A week after Dr. Purdy told me about the mass in my eye, I received a call from a friendly lady named Lee Penny from the Ocular Oncology Clinic in the Princess Margaret Hospital in Toronto. Lee told me I was scheduled to see the team of specialists for testing on June 8, and I would be getting my test results and diagnosis on June 10. She said if they needed to operate, it would likely take several weeks to be scheduled. When I hung up the phone, I immediately started feeling anxious, especially since my appointment was just two weeks away. Somehow, we had to get Matt, the pets, the house, and Gary's business ready for our absence, plus we had to get ourselves all the way to Toronto in time for my appointment.

The following day, I had an appointment with Dr. Purdy, the ophthalmologist. He said the pressure had come down so I could stop taking the pills and use the drops only. I was relieved as the pills lowered my blood pressure and made me feel tired and sick. I was hopeful I would feel better in time for our upcoming trip.

A couple of days later, I bought a lottery ticket. I knew I was likely just wasting my money, but it gave me some hope. Even though I knew I had to go to Toronto, I felt terrible I didn't have any savings to contribute and Gary would have to cover all of our expenses. I was also feeling anxious about missing so much time from work. I hadn't been back since Dr. Purdy told me about the mass and I had no idea when I would be able to return. I was working in customer service for a financial institution. It wasn't my preferred career as I had studied English literature in university and had hoped to become an editor, technical writer, or freelance writer, but those types of jobs were rare in my small city. I had settled for the most stable position I could find with a decent wage and full benefits.

Having so much time to myself gave me a chance to think about what I wanted to do with the rest of my life. *For all I know,* I kept thinking, *I might only have a few good years left.* I started thinking about what I would do if I could have my pick. I thought about earning a degree in performing arts, since I loved to act, dance, and sing. I also thought I would love to be a fashion designer, or an author. I wasn't sure if any of my ideas were even a remote possibility, but I realized I had to seriously consider my options before I ran out of time.

On June 2, 2004, with only two days left of high school, Matt turned eighteen years old. We had a low-key birthday celebration, but we made sure to pick up his favorite fully loaded pizza, a double chocolate cake, and a large container of ice cream. We bought him the new video game he had been wanting and one of his friends came over to hang out with him for the night. It was hard to believe how quickly the years had gone by, and that he had reached the age I was when he was born.

In November of 1985, just five months after I graduated from high school, I was working as a cashier in a pharmacy and trying to decide what to do with my life when I started feeling sick. I was vomiting multiple times each day and I was feeling dizzy and exhausted. My mother was concerned and questioned me every day about my symptoms. She had returned to her job as a secretary for the government after recovering from her mastectomy and chemotherapy treatments, but the cancer had changed her. She had dark circles under her eyes, low energy, and she rarely smiled. She spent a great deal of time alone in her bedroom and when she'd immerge, her eyes were often red and puffy. When I'd ask her if she was okay and if she'd been crying, she'd say she was just tired. One day, after I threw up yet again, she took me to the doctor to find out what was wrong with me. After a few tests, the doctor announced that I was three months pregnant. My mother gasped as tears welled up in her eyes. I was surprised and upset as well, I had been having my usual spotty periods and had thought I just had a stomach flu. On the way home from the doctor, my mother was silent in the car; I felt bad I was adding to her stress and unhappiness. Matt's birth father and I had a rocky relationship and had broken up a couple of months before, so I was not surprised when he said he did not want to be involved.

I had expected my pregnancy to cause some issues between my parents but since my mother's breast cancer, their fighting and arguing had been replaced by silence and avoidance, and this was no different. Eventually, we all embraced the idea of a new baby. My mother helped me pick out baby clothes and other necessary items, and my father transformed the downstairs of the house into a two-bedroom apartment. We furnished it with hand-me-downs and yard sale finds and installed some wallpaper with rainbows and puffy clouds in the nursery. Matt's birth was a challenge. My blood pressure skyrocketed, and I was unable to dilate beyond a couple of centimetres; after eighteen hours of labour, he was born via caesarean section. It was difficult to recover from my surgery while caring for an infant. My mother helped me as much as she could, but she was working full time and still struggling with her own issues.

After a couple of painful months, I was back to my old self but, there was a problem. Even though Matt was a big baby and had reached full term, he had a serious health issue. He frequently had croup (an infection that leads to swelling inside the trachea) and would have trouble breathing. By the time he reached eleven months old, the doctors discovered his trachea was not growing at a normal rate. They took him into surgery and put in a tracheotomy (an incision was made in his neck and a tube was placed into his windpipe). It was heartbreaking to watch my baby boy struggle to breathe and terrifying to have him operated on at such a young age. Fortunately, he recovered quickly and within a few days of his surgery, he was breathing normally and full of energy. A few weeks later, he was released from the hospital, however his tracheotomy would remain and every few months Matt would return to the hospital to have his windpipe stretched. It was a difficult time but despite his illness, he was a happy toddler and a joy to be around.

Six months later, my parents realized they could no longer afford their house and put it up for sale. The last couple of years had been hard on my parents financially. My mother had been out of work for over six months after her surgery, my father had resigned from his sales executive position and started a home renovation business, and then there was the added expense of supporting Matt and I. A few months later, when the house sold, my parents rented a two-bedroom apartment in a new building on the edge of the city for themselves and told me I would have to find my own place. I was nervous about living on my own for the first time and so far from my parents, but I couldn't afford to be in their building. I settled for an apartment across town in an older building on the city bus route.

Unfortunately, my parents would not be able to take our seven-year-old terrier, Westie, with them as their apartment did not allow pets. I wanted to take him with me but after several tearful conversations, my mother convinced me to let him go saying it would be too difficult for me to care for him and little Matt who still had his tracheotomy. My parents found a nice family to adopt Westie and even though it broke my heart, I said good-bye to our little buddy. I had to believe that he was well cared for and happy as anything else was just too difficult to bear.

By the time Matt turned two years old, we had settled into our new apartment and had met quite a few new neighbours and their young children. His windpipe had finally reached a normal size, so his tracheotomy was removed, and I started a full time job as a nanny for a nearby family with two children who agreed to let me bring Matt along to their house each day. The days were busy but, in the evenings, after Matt went to bed, I was lonely and having a hard time adjusting to being on my own.

CHAPTER 5

ROAD TRIP

In the days leading up to our trip to Toronto, Gary was finishing up some work for his business and setting it up so he could work remotely, and I kept myself busy from morning until night cleaning and organizing the house. Instead of focusing on what was happening, I would get lost cleaning out closets, doing loads and loads of laundry, and organizing and reorganizing everything in sight. I had convinced myself that if everything was clean and organized, everything would be okay. Unfortunately, no matter how busy I was, I could not shake the constant feeling of dread and every once in a while, I would feel a lump forming in my throat and have to take some deep breaths to avoid breaking down.

The day before we were scheduled to leave, Gary and I mapped out our 1,300-kilometre trip, highlighting the route and the highway numbers. I also made several lists—our itinerary, contact information, the pets' feeding instructions, and emergency numbers—and taped them onto the fridge. With the house cleaned and our bags packed, I could no longer ignore my feelings. I was worried about leaving Matt and the animals and I was nervous about our long road trip and being in an extremely large unfamiliar city.

That night, I had trouble sleeping. I couldn't avoid the fact that my ophthalmologist thought I should see the team of specialists in a Toronto cancer hospital. He didn't say it, but Dr. Purdy must have thought the mass was cancer. I couldn't help wondering, *If it is cancer, how long has it been there, and has it spread? Will I need chemotherapy or radiation or was it too late?* It was too scary to think about. I realized there was no point in speculating or worrying because within a few days I would know exactly what was wrong with my eye.

On June 7, 2004, Gary and I got up early, packed the car, went over the instructions for the pets with Matt, and left for Toronto. It had been over a decade since either of us had travelled any distance and we were excited to begin our adventure and spend some quality time together despite the reason for the trip. It was a typical spring day, and the weather changed from partly cloudy, to overcast, to rainy periods throughout our drive. I thoroughly enjoyed seeing the small towns and busy cities along the way, as well as the ever-changing landscape. As we crossed the border from Quebec into Ontario, the familiar sights, sounds, and smells reminded me of my childhood, and I suddenly felt like I was going home.

In the early 1960s, my parents left their family homes in Prince Edward Island (PEI) seeking employment. My mother lived with one of her sisters in Montreal, Quebec for several years while working in a hospital, and then moved in with another one of her sisters in Hamilton, Ontario and worked in a factory. My father spent a few years in the army before settling in Hamilton where he found work in a quarry. My parents met through friends, dated for a couple of months, and got married. Through upgrading their education and climbing the career ladder, my mother became a secretary and my father became a sales executive and they bought a little house in St. Catharines, Ontario. After nearly two decades in Ontario, they decided to move back to PEI, hoping to return to a simpler way of life and to be closer to family and friends. At eleven years old, I packed up my pretty pink bedroom, said goodbye to my friends and teachers at my Catholic school, and I hadn't been back since. Our family moved into a spacious house on a large lot in the small town of Stratford in rural PEI. It was a drastic change from the bustling city life in St. Catharines where I could walk to school, the local pool, and countless friends' houses. Summers in PEI were beautiful with breezy sunny days and white sandy beaches, but the harsh island winters were relentless with an endless string of snowstorms bringing high winds and frequent power outages. Winter wasn't my only issue as I was struggling in school; I didn't fit in well with my new schoolmates and was often bullied and excluded. After three years of island life, my father was offered a promotion so we pulled up stakes and moved to Fredericton, New Brunswick. I was sad to leave our extended family and the few friends I had made but Fredericton felt like a fresh start. Our new house was within walking distance of my new school, a variety of stores, a theatre, and it was on the city bus route, allowing me to have the independence I craved. I quickly made friends in my neighbourhood and at school where I joined the Art Club. There was trouble brewing at home though; the recent move had revealed cracks in my parent's marriage. Among other things, my mother was not happy about moving away from her friends and family and her new secretary job at an elementary school. This led to constant bickering and fighting. I was worried my parents were going to get a divorce and we would have to move again, but there was a much more serious problem that was about to reveal itself. Less than two years after moving to Fredericton, during a routine self-exam, my mother felt a large lump in her breast.

After fourteen long hours on the road stopping only for gas, food, and washroom breaks, Gary and I arrived in Toronto. I was overwhelmed by the crowds, noise, and steady traffic, and looking up at the tall buildings made me dizzy. We located the hotel in downtown Toronto and discovered the parking was underground. Being somewhat claustrophobic, I was uncomfortable with the prospect of going underground but we didn't have any other options. I cringed as the car dipped down into the dark, concrete structure. The low ceilings felt even lower due to the hanging yellow florescent lights and the labyrinth of exposed pipes. The roadways were barely wide enough for one car width, but Gary managed to safely maneuver the car and found a parking space near an elevator. The drive was exhausting, and we were both ready to check into our hotel room and rest.

Stepping off the elevator, I was immediately struck by the stunning hotel lobby. It had dark, polished wood floors, grand ceilings with sparkling chandeliers, enormous windows, and wide open spaces. The lobby was buzzing with staff in stiff uniforms and countless guests coming and going. I was suddenly excited about all the amazing things we would see while we were visiting the city. We checked into our room, ducked out for some takeout at a nearby restaurant, and settled in for the night.

CHAPTER 6

DISTURBING DIAGNOSIS

The next morning, we left the hotel and walked two blocks down the street to the Princess Margaret Hospital. The front of the hospital was an older six-story building with beige stone and small windows, but behind the facade it had a sleek, modern structure made of concrete and glass that shot up into the sky. We stepped into the elevator and went up to the Ocular Oncology Clinic on the eighteenth floor. The spacious clinic was bright and modern. I checked in with the receptionist, filled out some paperwork, and then we were directed to take a seat in the waiting room. The large waiting room had multiple windows overlooking the city and several rows of grey cushioned chairs; enough seating for at least thirty people.

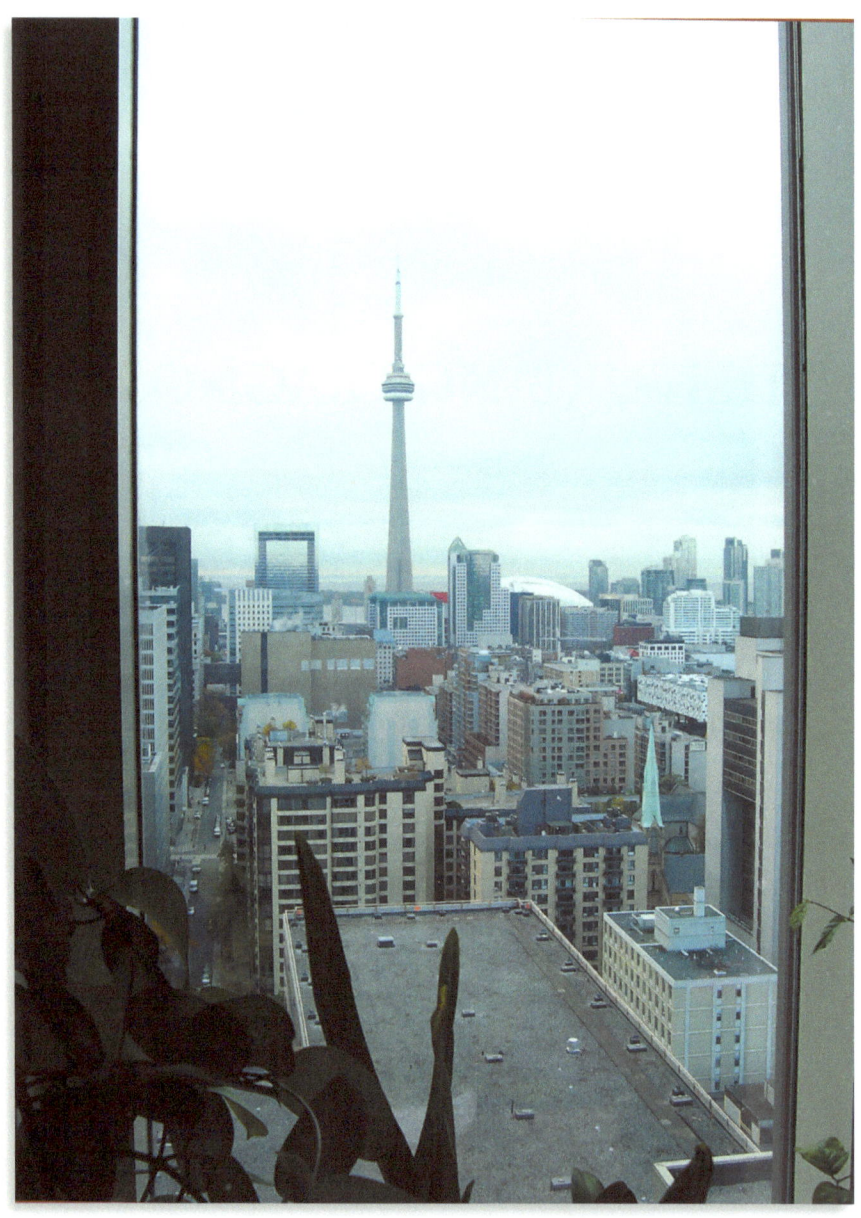

I took this picture from the waiting room of the Ocular Oncology Clinic in the Princess Margaret Hospital. June 8, 2004.

When my name was called, we followed a tall, middle aged doctor into an examination room. We exchanged pleasantries; the doctor was friendly and kind. He asked me to sit down and rest my chin on a little shelf attached to an eye testing device (slit lamp). He looked into my eye through the device, and then he suddenly pushed his chair back and looked at Gary. He leaned forward again, looked into my eye and sat back once again.

"If you have what I think you have, you may only have six months to live," he said with a serious look on his face.

I was in shock. *What was he was saying?* I felt fine and could not imagine for a moment I could die within six months. The doctor said he was quite certain I had iris melanoma, an extremely rare, highly lethal form of eye cancer that grows around the iris. Once it has grown all the way around the iris, it quickly spreads to the liver and throughout the body. My best chance for survival—if the cancer had not yet spread—was to remove my eye. He would run more tests to determine the stage of the cancer and also said I would need to have a blood test and chest X-rays. I asked him about plaque radiation therapy, but he quickly dismissed it saying that treatment was not for my type of tumour. A team of doctors would review my case and meet with me in two days to discuss the best course of action.

The doctor sent Gary back to the waiting room and took me into another examination room for an ultrasound of my eye. He put some drops into my eye to numb it for the test. It felt like getting soap in my eye, but after a couple of seconds my eye went numb and the pain was gone. He reclined my chair all the way back, placed what looked like a cup with no bottom directly on my eye, poured some solution into the cup, and pressed a long narrow wand against the surface of my eye. It was very strange as I could see the wand moving around in the solution, but I couldn't feel anything. Eventually, the numbing started to wear off and it became painful. The doctor said he could put more drops into my eye, but that he was almost finished. I told him to continue, hoping the pain wouldn't get much worse.

When it was finally over, I walked back into the waiting room, sat down beside Gary, buried my face in my hands and started to cry. Gary was worried and asked if the doctor had told me anything else. I told him he hadn't said anything, but the test was extremely painful, and I was completely exhausted and overwhelmed. Gary hugged me and reassured me it was almost over.

After a few more tests, we left the clinic and made our way to the lab for my blood test and X-rays. The chest X-rays were quick and painless but, because of my fear of needles, having my blood drawn made my anxiety level peak. We finally left the hospital, grabbed some food, and headed back to the hotel. After the day we had, all we wanted to do was shut the world out and relax.

That evening, I wrote the following in my journal:

> *Tuesday, June 8, 2004: Today was test day and was it ever rough! Three different doctors ran a whole slew of tests and it really sucked! Especially the ultrasound! So, the doctor said it is cancer and the entire eye must be removed! He also said it may have spread so they did chest X-rays and blood tests. We'll find out on Thursday.* [The] *doctor said the tumour is around the iris in a circle and other spots as well also, so it cannot be treated. Well, I guess we'll just deal with it!*

The next day was our free day in Toronto but it was 32°C and humid with a smog warning. Despite the heat and still being in shock about everything we were told the day before, we decided to venture out and explore the city. Our first stop was Casa Loma, a historical castle in midtown Toronto. The castle was beautiful and had a fascinating story, but it was difficult to enjoy because it was crowded and sweltering inside the building. Halfway through the tour, I lost my purse; I had tucked it behind a flower arrangement while Gary took my picture, then we walked away. By the time I realized it was missing, we were in the stables at the other end of the property. We ran through the fifty-foot-long underground tunnel all the way back to where I had left it. Thankfully, we found my purse untouched.

THE VIEW FROM MY WINDOW

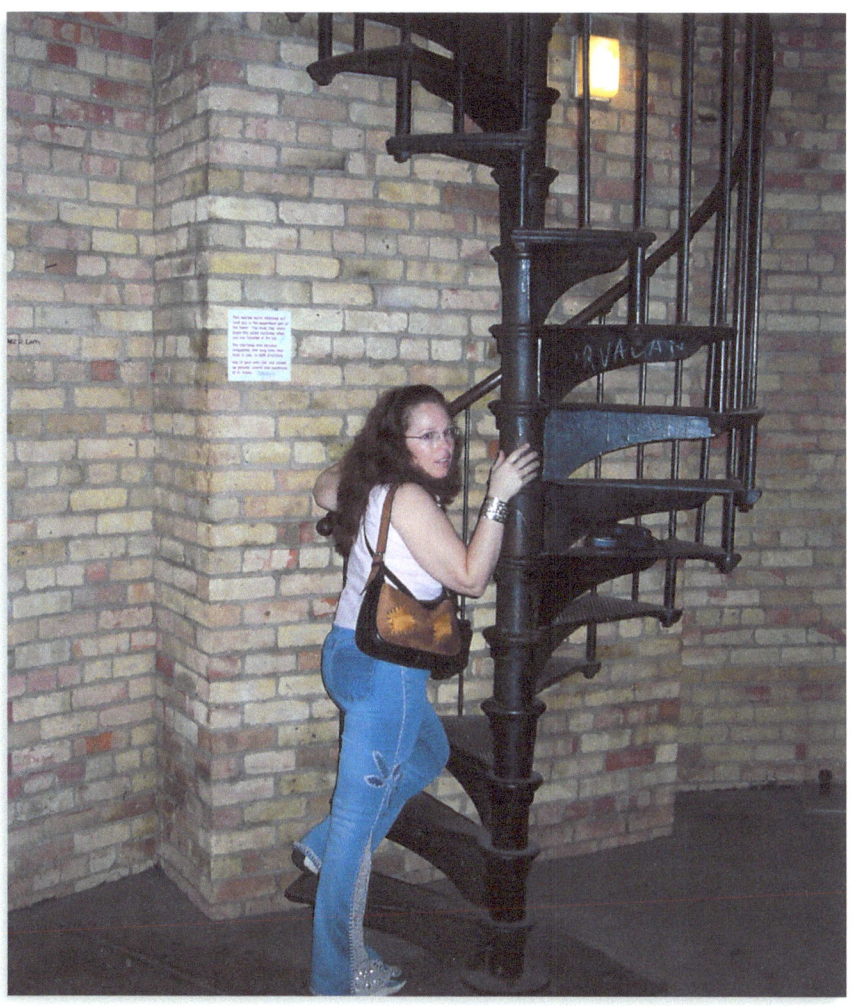

Gary took this picture of me inside Casa Loma after I found my purse. I was feeling hot and tired and not looking forward to climbing more stairs. June 9, 2004.

We left the castle and headed downtown to the CN Tower. Because of my fear of heights, I was nervous to go up in the tall tower, but I didn't want to miss the opportunity to experience such an amazing landmark. Standing on the observation deck looking at the view of the entire city was breathtaking, but it made me feel small; one of millions of people who may or may not survive. I tried to stay positive knowing I was being looked after by some of the best doctors in the world.

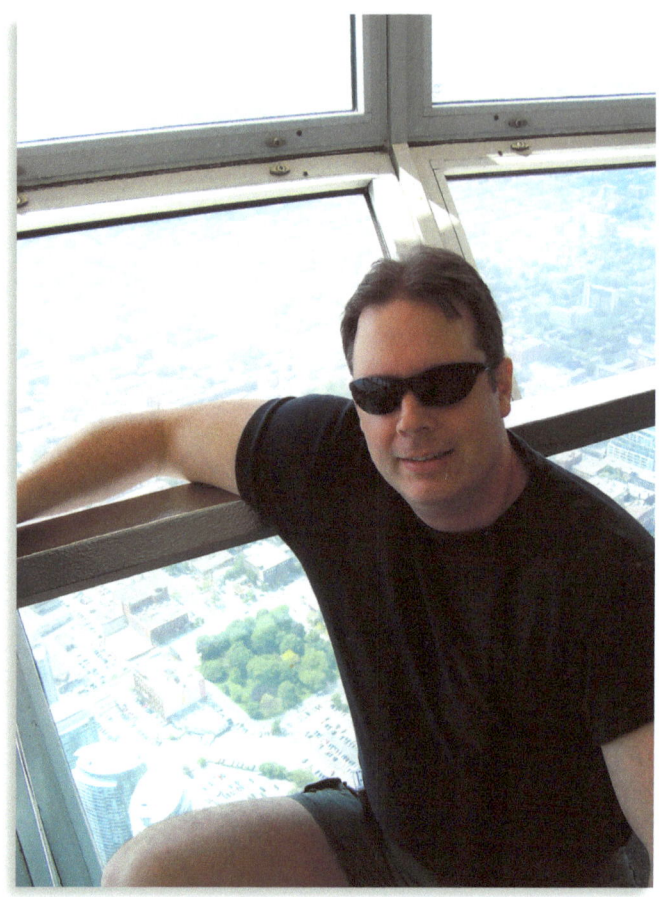

*I took this picture of my handsome fiancé,
Gary, while we were in the CN Tower.
June 9, 2004.*

We left the CN Tower and made our way back to the hotel to take a much-needed nap in our cool air-conditioned room. We woke up a few hours later and walked one block down the street to the Eaton Centre Mall. We wandered around the mall for a couple of hours; it was enormous and bright and had multiple floors full of stunning shops with beautiful items. As we were walking past one of the clothing stores, I was drawn in by its unique style. Inside the changing room, I looked at myself in the mirror while contemplating a black and pink asymmetrical blouse. Despite what I was going through, I still looked the same. I still had the same long, wavy brown hair, big blue eyes, and freckles, but my midsection was soft from too many missed workouts, and there was a sadness in my face. I shrugged it off knowing I had much bigger issues to deal with and stepped out of the changing room to model the new top for Gary. Despite being tired, overwhelmed, and nervous about my uncertain future, we did our best to stay in the moment and had a fun and exciting day.

We got up early the next morning and went back to the clinic. While we were in the waiting room, an elderly gentleman and his family came out of an examination room. The man looked tired and frail. His daughter was pacing and talking on her cell phone; she was telling someone nothing could be done to help her father as his cancer had spread. They were visibly distraught. They all left, and Gary and I were once again alone in the waiting room. I told Gary that my worst fear was the doctors telling me they couldn't help me. He tried to reassure me; he said I was young and strong and could fight anything thrown my way. I appreciated his positivity, but we both knew if the cancer had spread to my liver, I would not survive.

I was surprised to be called into the examination room again as I thought the day was only about test results and treatment options. I didn't question it, though, and walked into the small windowless room with the hope they wouldn't be doing anything painful. The doctor asked me to sit down and, once again, rest my chin on the little shelf attached to the slit lamp. He looked at my eye through the device, and then he said the Princess Margaret Hospital was a teaching hospital and asked if I would allow some medical students to come in and look at my eye. I gave my permission and several young students in long white lab coats quietly came in and, one by one, looked at my eye. As strange as it was to be a spectacle for the students, I didn't mind if it meant helping them diagnose their future patients. I walked back out to the waiting room, sat down beside Gary, and waited for the doctors to call me.

My name was called again, and Gary and I walked into a large, white, clinical room. A few minutes later, several doctors came in and sat down. Dr. McGowan introduced himself and advised us he would be handling my case. He was a tall, thin, middle aged man with dark hair, a tidy moustache, and a serious demeanour. He introduced the other doctors in the room and then said there was a 99% chance the growth in my eye was cancer. He mentioned a biopsy was not an option because it could cause the cancer to spread. Dr. McGowan said I had iris melanoma. He echoed what the first doctor told us two days prior, describing it as a fast-growing cancer. If it was to spread beyond my eye, he confirmed I would have less than six months to live. He said the test showed the cancer had not yet grown all the way around my iris, but the only way to prevent the cancer from spreading was to remove my eye.

I think the doctor was expecting me to gasp or cry or something, but instead I just nodded and asked when he would be able to operate. He was surprised by my lack of reaction and asked if I understood I had cancer and my eye had to be removed. Gary told Dr. McGowan we had already determined I would end up losing my eye based on the information we were given during my tests. Even though I wasn't surprised, I did feel sad and nervous about losing my eye and having to go through such an invasive surgery.

I was surprised when Dr. McGowan told me he could operate the following week. As much as I wanted to get rid of the cancer, there was a problem: Matt's high school graduation ceremony was the following week. I asked the doctor if it would be safe to delay the surgery for a few weeks. I was told as long as I continued to be monitored by my ophthalmologist to keep the pressure down in my eye, I should be fine. I was relieved; I would have been crushed if I wasn't able to attend Matt's graduation ceremony.

Dr. McGowan then explained what the enucleation (eye removal) and orbital implant surgery involved. My eye would be removed but the muscles and the rest of the orbital contents would remain intact. A porous orbital implant would be covered with donor sclera (eye) tissue and attached to some of my optic muscles. This would enable my new eye to move naturally. Once I recovered from the surgery, a prosthetic eye would be made to fit in front of the implant. I was given some articles and pamphlets about the surgery and told I would be contacted with a surgery date. One of the pamphlets described the surgery and had a detailed drawing of an implant and the attached muscles. The whole process looked and sounded intricate and complex; all I could do was hope the doctors knew what they were doing.

As the meeting seemed to be coming to a close, Gary asked Dr. McGowan about the results of my blood test and chest X-rays. He didn't have the information with him, so he sent us back out to the waiting room while he checked my test results. Gary and I quietly walked hand in hand back out to the waiting room and sat down. A few minutes later one of the other doctors came over to us and, as I had expected, he said there wasn't any evidence of cancer in my blood or my lungs. Gary was so relieved when he heard the news, he broke down. It was heart wrenching to see him so upset. This whole experience had been overwhelming for him as well, and from what the doctors said the day of my tests, he was convinced the cancer had spread and I wouldn't live much longer. Walking out of the hospital, Gary was grateful I would live, and I was horrified I was going to lose my eye. Back at the hotel, we quickly packed our things, brought them down to the car and headed for home.

CHAPTER 7

MAKING TIME FOR METAL

We drove all night and arrived home around 8:00 a.m. Gary and I both felt a sense of relief as we pulled into our driveway. Jody, Kitty, and Matt were glad to see us. We unpacked the car and settled back in. Within a few hours of being home, I received a phone call from a woman from work in human resources. She was wondering about my status and if I had any updates for her. I told her I had just found out I had cancer and was going to lose my eye. She was very kind and empathetic, but her call felt somewhat intrusive since Gary and I hadn't yet had a chance to share the news with anyone. That evening we contacted our family and friends and explained my situation. It was shocking news, but we did our best to explain the complex surgery and my new prosthetic eye even though we had a thin grasp on the details and what was about to happen to me.

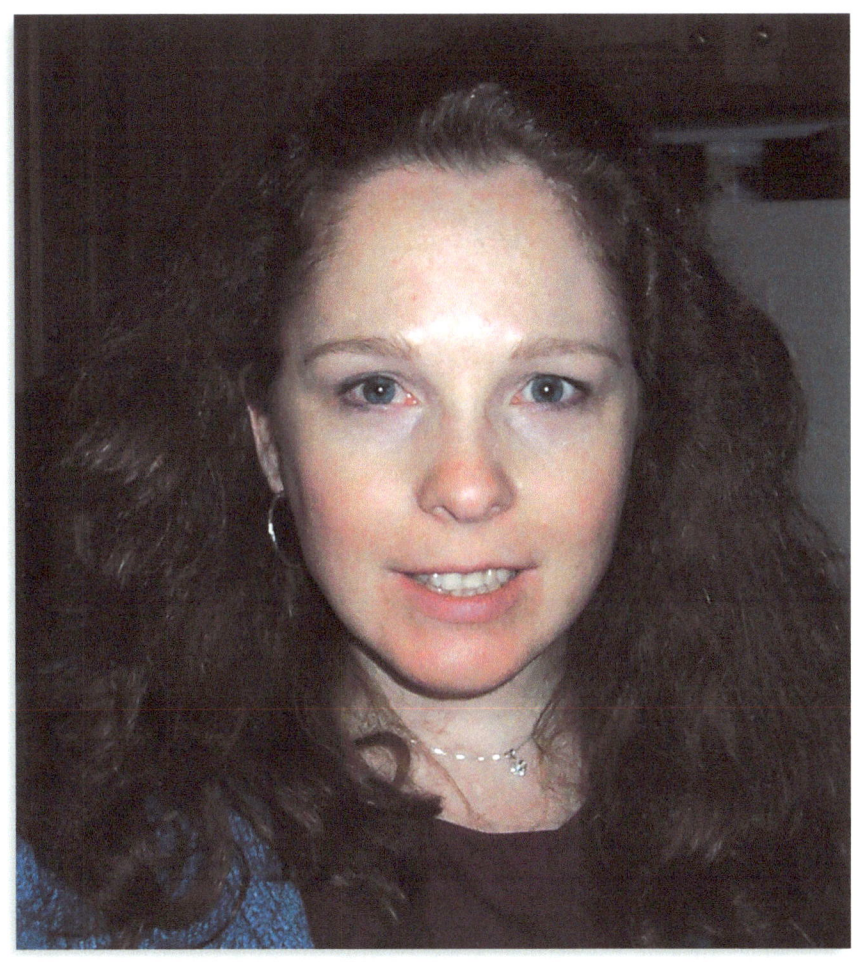

*I asked Gary to take a few pictures when we got home.
This is one of the last pictures taken before I lost my eye to cancer.
June 11, 2004.*

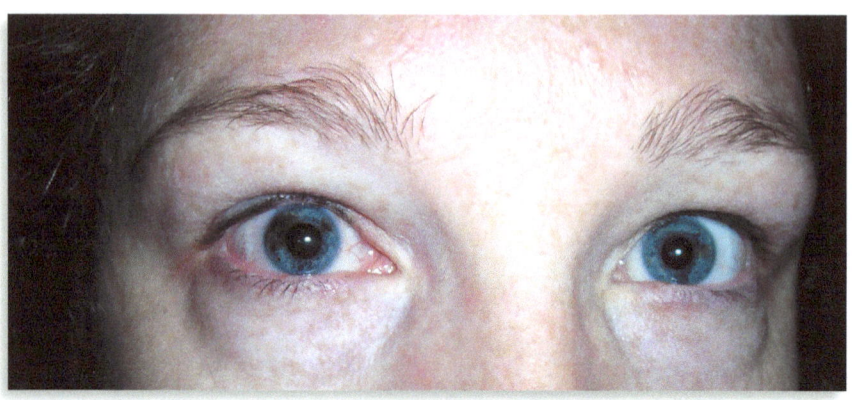

A close-up picture of my eyes. The pupil in my right eye is misshapen and the dark area in the iris is the tumour. My eye was bloodshot due to glaucoma and a detached retina. June 11, 2004.

The next day, Gary and I and a couple of our friends drove to St. John, New Brunswick to watch a performance of one of Gary's favorite bands, Slayer. We had bought our tickets several months prior to my eye issues, and we thought it would be a good distraction from our harsh reality. We met a couple more of our friends at the coliseum and we were all looking forward to the concert. It was comforting to be with our friends; everyone was concerned and encouraging, but I was still feeling a little shaken by my recent diagnosis. By the time we were heading to our seats, the concert had already started so it was loud and dark inside the arena. Because of my glaucoma and detached retina, I found it difficult to see in the dark, and I was nervous about going down the steep concrete stairs. Gary held my hand and led me to my seat. I was thankful for his help, but it made me realize I was going to need a lot of help while I adjusted to my new single-eye life. We enjoyed the concert, and I tried my best not to think about it being the last concert I would see with two eyes.

The next afternoon, I was looking over the pamphlets and articles Dr. McGowan had given me. One of them mentioned preparing for single-eye vision by covering my eye for a few minutes or hours each day leading up to my surgery. It recommended using either an eyepatch or taping a tissue over my eyeglass's lens. After my first attempt at patching my eye for an hour, I had a headache and felt nauseated. I didn't give up, though, and continued to patch my eye for at least an hour every day to help me ease into single-eye vision.

Patching my eye gave me an idea. Since it would be at least six weeks after surgery before I would be fitted for my prosthetic eye, I decided to make some custom eyepatches designed to match my clothing. That evening while Gary and I were running errands, we stopped at a fabric store and bought some supplies to make eyepatches. I picked out some bright and colourful fabric and several metres of elastic. I had always enjoyed being creative, and I was excited to work on this fun and productive project.

CHAPTER 8

OUR GRADUATE

A week later, Gary, his mother, Muriel, and I climbed up the steep bleacher stairs of Matt's high school auditorium. The large room was crowded and noisy with an air of excitement. We found some empty seats with a clear view of the stage and sat down. It was difficult to believe that just one week prior, I was in Toronto being told I had cancer and might die within six months. I tried to push away my negative thoughts and focus on Matt's graduation ceremony.

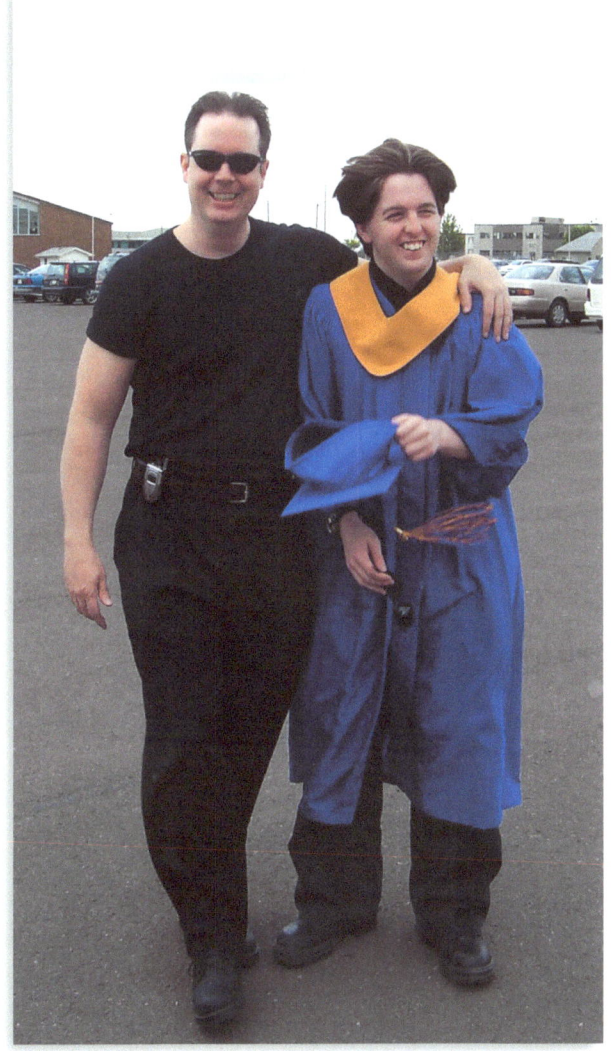

Proud Dad and Matt goofing off on graduation day while walking into the auditorium. June 17, 2004.

Tears filled my eyes as I stood with the rest of the spectators to watch the nearly 200 graduates enter the auditorium. All eyes were on the graduates as they marched in two by two each wearing a traditional graduation cap and gown. After several inspirational speeches, the students lined up and took turns walking across the stage. When it was Matt's turn, Gary squeezed my hand as I fought back tears. We beamed with pride as we watched Matt accept his diploma. It was a heartwarming experience, and I was grateful I was able to attend such an important milestone in our son's life.

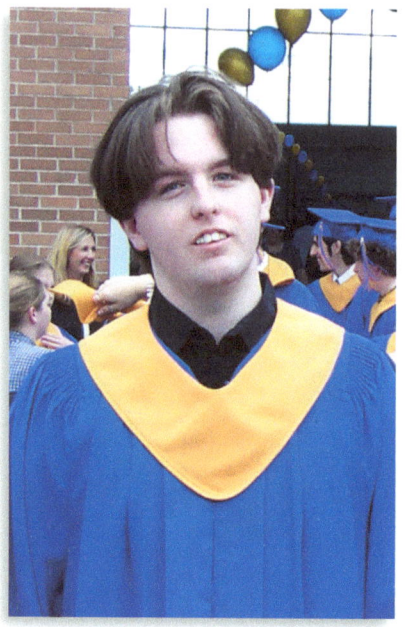

Matt outside after the ceremony with the other graduates. June 17, 2004.

I was so proud of Matt. Despite his rocky start in life, he had excelled in school. He enjoyed learning, easily picked up new concepts and information, always finished his work on time, and got along well with his classmates and teachers. Even though he had mapped out some long-term plans, he decided to take a gap year before starting university. We supported his decision as long as he worked full time.

Matt quickly found a job stocking shelves overnight at a local department store. It was strange not to have him home at night, but I had to accept that my little boy was growing up. Before long, Gary and I would be returning to Toronto for my surgery and we would be away from him for over a week. I had to let go and hope he would be okay.

CHAPTER 9

THE WAITING PERIOD

During June and July, our house was chaotic and busy. We were finishing up some renovations we had planned prior to my eye issues. We ordered new steel doors and casement grill windows, and we were painting the exterior of the house beige with white trim. I had intended to help Gary paint the house, but since I was instructed by the doctors to take it easy, Gary took the lead and I only helped when I was feeling up to it.

One day near the end of June, I was having a really good day. I was outside working in the back garden and enjoying the summer weather. I was feeling so healthy and normal that I couldn't believe three weeks earlier I was in Toronto being told I had cancer. Suddenly, Gary was at the door telling me the phone was for me. It was Dr. McGowan's receptionist calling to book my surgery date. My heart pounded as I took down her instructions. I thanked her for the information and hung up the phone as a wave of dread washed over me. With my eye removal surgery just one month away, I could no longer live in denial. I had to face the facts: my surgery was coming, and this would be my last summer with two eyes.

Around this time, I went to see my family doctor, Dr. Dempsey. I wanted to have a few lumps on my neck looked at, and I wanted a prescription for an anti-anxiety medication. I had noticed the lumps awhile back, but I didn't think much about them until the Toronto doctors told me I had cancer. She examined the lumps and told me they were likely nothing to worry about, but I should check them monthly and contact her if they started to grow. Knowing about my mother's history, she also reminded me to continue to do regular breast exams and watch for anything else unusual. She gave me a prescription for an anti-anxiety medication. I had taken the medication previously so I knew it would be helpful. As my operation approached, my anxiety was building, and I wanted to be prepared in case I ended up having a breakdown in Toronto. Dr. Dempsey was kind and attentive and asked me a few questions about my eye surgery. She wished me luck with everything and told me to contact her if I needed anything.

The following is the journal entry I wrote the day after my doctor's appointment.

> *Thursday, June 24, 2004: When I was at the doctor's office, she looked at me with such sympathy in her eyes that I felt sad. It's so weird how that works but I'm perfectly fine right up until someone says "Oh you poor thing," even if it's just with their actions.*

Our new front door was installed during the first week of July. It had multiple raised panels and a small leaded glass window. It was vast improvement from the warped, cracked, wooden door it replaced. I was excited to paint it navy blue, as soon as the installer left, I grabbed my paint supplies, propped the door open, and started painting. Suddenly, out of nowhere, there was a clap of thunder and my dog, Jody, who had been sleeping on the living room couch, got scared and ran out the open door. Jody was well trained and would normally listen to commands off leash, but she was afraid of the thunder and refused to stop when I called out to her. I grabbed my shoes and ran after her, but she was running so fast she was out of my sight within a couple of seconds. I ran around the neighbourhood frantically searching for my sweet dog, but I couldn't find her anywhere and she wouldn't come to my repeated calls for her.

I raced back home and told Gary and Matt. They got into the car and drove around the neighbourhood looking for her while I went out again on foot. A few minutes later, the sky opened and a downpour erupted. I was worried someone would try to approach Jody and she would bite them out of fear. I was desperate to find her before anything happened. After a couple more unsuccessful laps around the block, I was cold and soaking wet and headed back toward the house with the hope Gary and Matt had found her. I was in tears and feeling defeated when I spotted my poor girl drenched and shaking on the front step of our house. I brought her in and dried her off. I was so relieved and thankful she was home safe and sound. I got Jody when she was just eight weeks old and she had been by my side ever since. She was my little pal, always keeping me company and making me feel loved and protected. It would have completely destroyed me if anything had happened to her.

I continued to have weekly appointments with Dr. Purdy to monitor the pressure in my eye. When I saw him on July 2, 2004, he noticed the pressure was building again so he prescribed a new medication (APO-Methazolamide 50MG). I knew the medication was necessary, but I was disappointed because the previous pills made me feel dizzy, tired, and nauseated, and I was certain these pills would have the same effect. While I was there, I decided to ask the doctor if I would be a candidate for laser eye surgery on my remaining eye. I had been wearing contact lenses for over fifteen years, and I thought it would be great if I never had to wear them or glasses ever again. He told me laser eye surgery was not an option because if something went wrong, I would be blind, and I should never wear contact lenses again because of the possibility of an infection. He also said since I'd lose my depth perception after my eye was removed, wearing glasses at all times was necessary to protect my remaining eye from projectiles and accidents. I was disappointed but I certainly didn't want to end up blind. I knew I had to be responsible and protect my remaining eye.

CHAPTER 10

BACK TO TORONTO

P lanning our return trip to Toronto was a bit more complicated this time as Gary and I would be gone for ten days. Dr. McGowan recommended I stay in the city for seven days following the surgery; he wanted to be close by in case I had any complications. Gary was busy getting prepared as he would again be working remotely while we were away, and I was back to my old tricks: cleaning, organizing and making lists; anything to avoid dealing my feelings of dread. Gary's mother, Muriel, offered to help Matt look after the animals, the house, and pick up groceries. We were grateful for her help since we didn't want to put too much pressure on Matt. From my own experience with my mother's cancer, I knew all too well how stressful this whole situation could be for him.

The following is the journal entry I wrote during this time when I was feeling exceptionally frustrated.

> *Wednesday, July 14, 2004: Anger is a very interesting emotion. What I've noticed is that because I'm very angry right now, everything else makes me steaming mad! Gary has gotten used to my frequent outbursts of anger. They're not directed at him, but just in general. Say something on the news…and I'm off on a rage.*

> *… I had two strange dreams last night. In one dream somehow, I got nail polish on my good eye and I was very distressed it would ruin my vision and I would be blind. In the second dream, I heard a baby crying while I was walking outside, and I found a baby in a covered ditch. She was okay but it was pretty disturbing.*

The following day, I was still struggling and wrote in my journal about my fear of hospitals seeking comfort from my mother.

> *Thursday, July 15, 2004: I hate that I have to stay two nights in the hospital. I hate hospitals. They stress me out! Oh well, this is just something I have to deal with and then I can get on with the rest of my life. Not everything in life is pleasant, as a matter of fact most things are not, it's how we can see the good.* [I could hear my mom's words:] *"Remember sometimes* [bad] *things happen and it's not your fault. They just happen. Remember that you are a good girl and I will always love you." Mom, I really wish you were here right now. I know you would worry and stress out, but you always made me feel like I was going to be okay.*

The night before we left, I was feeling anxious about being away from our son and our pets for so long. At his age, Matt didn't mind having the place to himself for a while, but I was worried he would eventually get lonely. I was also worried about Jody and Kitty as I knew they wouldn't understand; it broke my heart to think about them being sad and lonely. I had to somehow put my feelings aside because I knew I had to go, and worrying wasn't going to change anything. I was a little nervous about my operation, but I was tired of waiting; it had been six weeks since I found out I had cancer, and I wanted to get rid of it before it spread.

The next morning, we got up early, packed the car and, once again, left for Toronto. It was the end of July, and this time we were fortunate enough to be traveling on a bright, sunny day. The scenery through Quebec was breathtaking. I was in awe of the majestic snow-capped mountains, the rolling fields of emerald green grass, and the array of colourful flowers scattered across the countryside. I'd always loved the beauty of nature, and I was grateful for the opportunity to experience the scenery one more time before I lost my eye. I tried to soak it all in, hoping to imprint my memory with the spectacular scenic views. I couldn't imagine how my vision would change after my surgery, but I was certain the world would never again look as beautiful as it did that day.

It was a long, exhausting trip, but we eventually made it back to the same downtown hotel we stayed at previously, and we checked in. As scary as it was to be diagnosed with cancer and facing surgery, I enjoyed being back in Toronto with Gary on yet another adventure. Even though we were painfully aware of our reality, we did our best to enjoy every moment together.

The next morning, we drove to Dr. McGowan's office in North York. We walked into the single-story concrete building, and I introduced myself to Dr. McGowan's receptionist. She handed me a clipboard and some papers to fill out. As I wrote Gary's information in the section for next of kin, I felt so grateful to have him by my side protecting me, guiding me, and supporting me at a time I felt the most vulnerable and afraid. I handed the paperwork back, and the receptionist advised me to go to the North York General Hospital for my pre-surgery tests.

At first glance, the large concrete hospital gave me mixed feelings of fear and appreciation. I was grateful my cancer was found and would be removed, but I was afraid of the recovery period and how my life would change afterwards. We walked into the building, checked in and were directed down a long hallway. My tests included checking my blood pressure, a cardiogram, and my least favourite, a blood test. When the tests were finished, I was free to leave, but I was instructed to be back by 6:30 a.m. the following morning. We enjoyed the rest of the day, did some shopping, went out to dinner at one of our favourite restaurants, and then went back to the hotel to watch a movie. We did our best to avoid the subject of my surgery; instead we tried to stay in the moment and enjoy each other's company.

CHAPTER 11

LIFE-ALTERING SURGERY

On July 29, 2004, I woke up at 5:00 a.m. thinking, *What if they're wrong? What if they made a mistake and it isn't cancer?*

I showered, got dressed, and packed. I could not believe what was about to happen; I was going to allow someone to remove my eye. It seemed crazy. I was also worried about living the rest of my life with only one eye. *Will I be able to adjust? Will I lose my independence?* I tried to push all of these thoughts and questions out of my mind; regardless of the doubts I was having, I wanted to live. I was certain my best chance for survival was to trust the specialists and let them remove my eye.

We drove up Yonge Street at 6:00 a.m. The sun was coming up and it was going to be a beautiful sunny day. The normally busy city streets were eerily quiet with very few people and very little traffic. Since I was fasting and I couldn't have any coffee, I was feeling tired and groggy. I was also feeling sad as Gary and I had been enjoying spending time together experiencing the city, and the fun part of our trip was over. I was not looking forward to the next couple of days, but I was hopeful I would recover quickly.

I checked into the North York General Hospital and was immediately taken into a small changing room. I was instructed to remove all of my clothing and jewelry, put on a hospital gown, a housecoat, and a pair of disposable medical booties. I had left my jewelry at the hotel; it was the first time I had taken off my engagement ring since Gary proposed, and I felt sad not to have it on. Until that point, I hadn't realized how much comfort my personal items gave me. After getting changed, I went back into the waiting room and sat down beside Gary. He held my hand as we quietly waited.

When my name was called, I got up and walked down the hallway with a nurse, but then I realized I was still wearing my glasses. I quickly went back into the waiting room and gave them to Gary. We said our goodbyes again, and I went back to find the nurse. She led me into a small white room and asked me to lie down on a gurney. She told me she was going to put an IV in the back of my hand. At the mention of an IV I could feel myself getting flushed as my heart started to race, but I knew it was necessary and the least of my concerns. I tried to focus on my breathing and looked away while she inserted the needle. Afterwards, the nurse wheeled my gurney into a long, bright hallway. She pushed my bed up against a large window, said the doctor would be with me shortly and walked away.

The sunshine was flooding in through the window; my limited vision was washed out by the brightness. I knew there was someone on a gurney behind me because I could hear rustling and an occasional cough. I wanted to tell them what was about to happen to me and ask them if they were going through the same type of thing, but I thought the person might be trying to rest, so I remained quiet. It felt like I waited for quite a while, at least twenty or thirty minutes. It was a really long time to be without my glasses, and I wondered if it was a mistake not to keep them with me. I closed my eyes and kept reminding myself this would all be over soon.

Finally, Dr. McGowan appeared and told me he was going to wheel me into surgery. I was comforted to see his familiar face, and I was confident he would take excellent care of me. From what I could see, the operating room was quite small with just a few feet for the doctor to move around.

With a hospital this large, I expected to be in a huge operating room with a team of doctors and nurses. Dr. McGowan told me he was going to remove my eye and put an implant in its place. I reminded him my right eye was the right eye to remove. I was terrified the wrong eye would be removed or I would somehow lose the sight in my good eye. He said he would be examining my eye before he operated. Some medication was injected into my IV, and I fell asleep.

The next thing I knew, I woke up in the recovery room. I had been in surgery for an hour and in the recovery room for an hour and a half.

I immediately tried to open my left eye (the good one), and to my great relief, I could still see. My vision was blurry, but I could see the shape of someone in white walking around the huge white recovery room. I closed my eye, put my hand to my face, and I could feel a large, protruding bandage over what was my right eye. The bandage forced my right eyelid to remain tightly closed, which made it difficult to fully open my left eye. I was relieved the operation was over and I wasn't feeling any pain.

The nurse must have seen me stirring because she came over, checked my vitals, and asked me a few general questions. She returned a few minutes later with a banana-flavoured popsicle. The cold popsicle was sweet and soothing on my dry throat. After I finished, the nurse decided it was time for me to go back to my room. On the way back, there were many twists and turns, including a jolting elevator ride, and I started feeling nauseated. I was only back in my room for a few minutes when I started to vomit. I continued to vomit on and off for the rest of the day. I was given several types of anti-nausea medication, but nothing seemed to make my stomach calm down until I was given an IV medication used for chemotherapy patients. I was exhausted, and Gary felt helpless watching me suffer. I was thankful to have him by my side bringing me whatever I needed or just keeping me company. With the help of the anti-nausea medication, I was able to sleep through the night.

The next morning, I woke up early. I could hear the sounds of the nurses changing shift and checking on patients. I was feeling groggy and I could barely see, but I was hungry. After the horrible day I had the day before, I knew having an appetite was a good sign, but it was still at least an hour before breakfast. I pulled open the top drawer of my nightstand and found the energy bar I had brought with me. I ate it and my stomach felt much better. I was feeling okay otherwise, but there was a great deal of pressure under the bandage and any movement of my left eye (the good one) would cause a sharp jolt of pain deep inside my right eye socket. I also needed to use the washroom, so I pushed my call button and a nurse came into my room. I tried to put on my glasses, but the bandage was so large that the arm of my glasses couldn't reach my right ear. The nurse used some medical tape to fasten the lens of my glasses to my eye bandage. It looked a little odd, but it worked, and it was certainly better than going without them. She helped me and my IV pole walk to the washroom and back. Afterwards, I told her about the pain in my eye socket; she injected some medication into my IV, and I was able to sleep for a few more hours.

When I woke up again, I was looking around the room and noticed something a little strange. It was difficult to describe, but I could see flashes of light and dark shadows over everything. I didn't understand what I was seeing, but it was as if I stared at a light too long and the traces of light remained after I looked away. I tried not to think about it too much and hoped it was only temporary. I looked on the top of my nightstand and saw a sheet of paper with a phone number written in giant numbers and the instructions to "Call Gary." I dialled the number and Gary immediately answered. He was relieved to hear my voice and not a nurse or doctor telling him something was wrong. I told him I was doing okay and asked him to pick me up a coffee and a muffin on his way to the hospital. He gladly complied, saying he was on his way.

Later that morning after Gary arrived, the nurse came in, checked my vitals, and removed my IV.

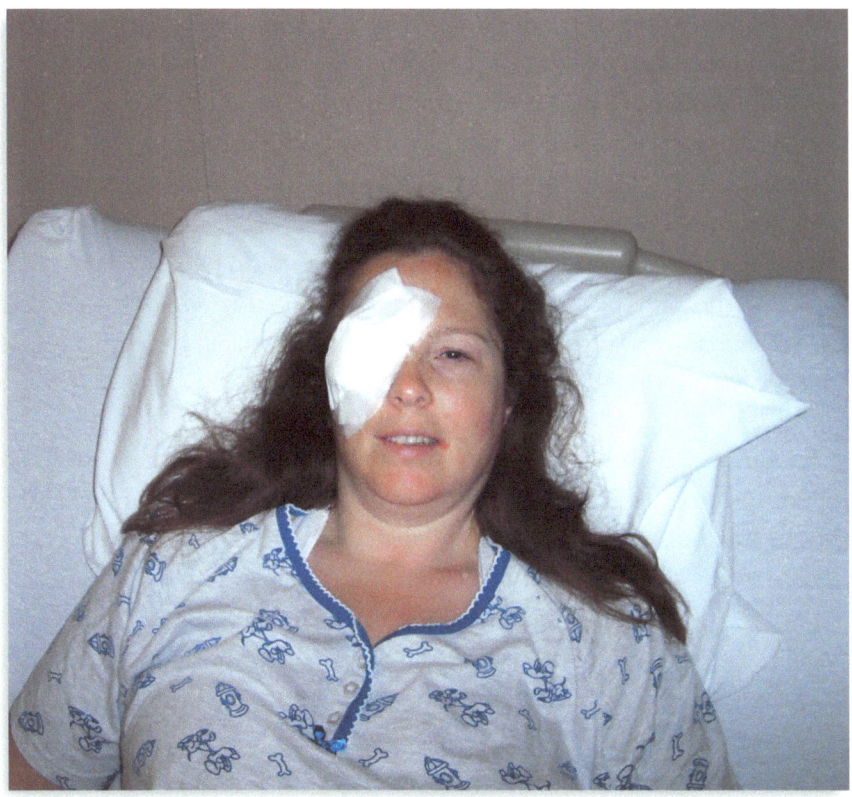

When the nurse left the room, Gary snapped this picture of me. July 30, 2004.

Shortly afterwards, Dr. McGowan came in to check on my progress and examine his work. He carefully pulled back the tape and lifted the large gauze bandage off of my new eye. It was extremely tight, so it was a great relief to have it off. I looked at Gary's face for a reaction but he remained stoic. Dr. McGowan cleaned around my new eye with a gauze pad and saline solution. He put some ointment between my eyelids and replaced my bandage with a thin, oval, cotton eye pad held in place with a single piece of medical tape. During the day I was to leave my new eye open to the air, and at night I was to apply some ointment and cover it with an eye pad. Dr. McGowan gave me several eye pads, a small tube of ointment (Tobradex), and a roll of medical tape. He told me to hold a cold facecloth on my new eye for ten minutes, three times per day. He also gave me a prescription for some pain medication to use as needed (Tylenol No. 2, Acetaminophen/Codeine Compound 15MG JNO).

Dr. McGowan said everything looked fine and, since I was eating normally, he would discharge me from the hospital. I was given an appointment to see him in one week before we went back home, but I was to contact him in the meantime if I had any issues. I told him about the pain I was feeling when I tried to look around. He said he had cut the optic muscles that were attached to my old eye and sewn them onto the tissue covering my new orbital implant. Any movement of my new eye would pull on the stitches. To avoid the pain, he recommended I move my head and not my eye. He also mentioned it was common to be dizzy and nauseated after eye removal surgery but, in time, I would adjust.

After the doctor left, I immediately went to look at my face in the washroom mirror. I carefully pulled back the tape and the eye pad. My eyelids were bright red and swollen but still fully intact. I could barely open my eyelid due to the swelling, but what I could see was a shiny red eye. The doctor had placed a clear acrylic conformer over my implant to ensure it would heal in the proper shape. This was my new reality. I was hopeful I would look very close to my original self once the swelling and bruising was gone and I was fitted with my prosthetic eye.

Gary helped me get dressed and pack my things. I was feeling dizzy and disoriented so he held my hand to steady me as we walked through the halls of the hospital. I realized I couldn't see very well; everything looked grey and foggy. I assumed I was still feeling the effects of the surgery and the pain medication. We got into the car and headed toward the hotel. Being in the car made me feel nauseated, so I leaned my seat back and tried to rest for the duration of the drive.

When my mother was discharged from the hospital after her mastectomy, I was excited and insisted on coming along. I had hoped she would come home, and everything would go back to normal, but as my father drove us away from the hospital, I realized things were far from normal. She was exceptionally nervous and irritated; she kept her hand on the dashboard and reacted with a gasp every time another car got close to us. On the way home, we stopped at our local pharmacy so my father could pick up her prescription and things escalated. While my mother and I waited in the car, she saw some young men standing outside of the store and she became extremely agitated and concerned. She was certain we were in danger and nothing I could say would calm her down. I was surprised by her paranoia and fear as she had always been strong and brave in every situation. Before long, my father came out of the pharmacy and drove us home. I realized my mother had been profoundly affected by her surgery, and I felt an overwhelming need to protect and comfort her.

When Gary and I arrived back at the hotel, I ate some oatmeal to settle my stomach and fell asleep. The next morning, I woke up at 4:00 a.m. feeling nauseated. I vomited several times over the next few hours. After taking some anti-nausea medication and drinking some ginger ale, I started to feel better. We were concerned the pain medication (codeine) might be making me sick as I had always had a poor reaction to any strong medication. From that point on, I only used acetaminophen for pain, and the nausea went away.

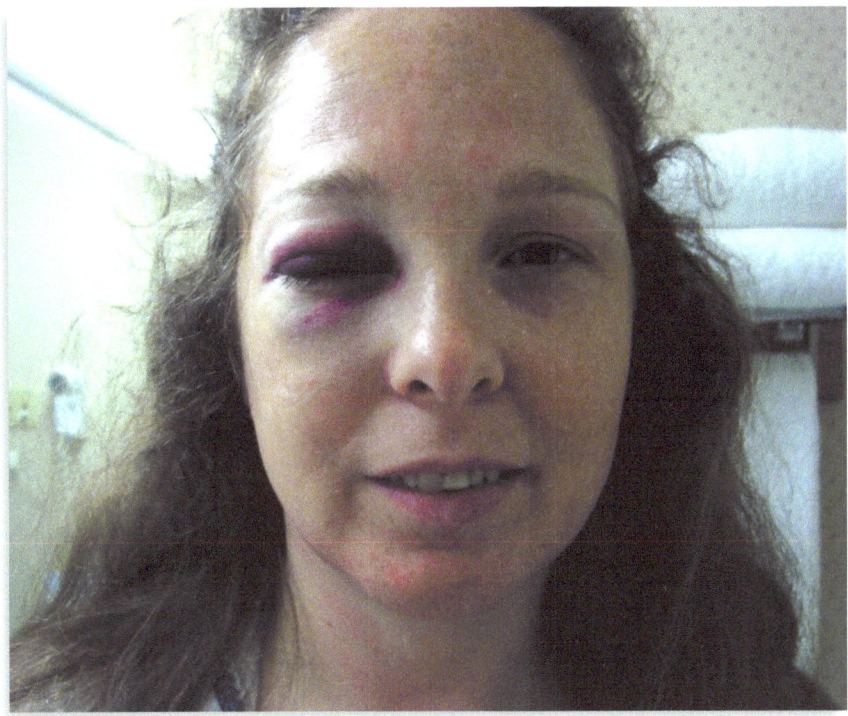

Gary took this picture at the hotel. July 31, 2004.

To bring down the swelling, Dr. McGowan recommended I hold a cold facecloth on my new eye, but I decided to take it one step further and use an ice pack. I made my own by filling a Ziplock bag with crushed ice and wrapping it in a clean, damp facecloth. I would lie down, propped up with a few pillows and place the ice pack on my eye and the surrounding area. I applied the ice pack at twenty-minute intervals: twenty minutes on/twenty minutes off. It was soothing on my wounded face and helped keep my pain under control.

The following is an email I sent out to our friends and family to update them on my progress.

> *Sunday, August 1, 2004: I just wanted to let you know that I am doing great! My surgery was on Thursday past and I was released from the hospital the next day. I have been slowly improving ever since. Gary has become my most fabulous nurse and I have been watching a lot of TV, putting a lot of ice on my head and just taking it easy. All is okay and I am feeling pretty good now. I had a few days where I felt like a complete bag of shit but that was to be expected. I have a seriously black eye that was swollen shut to begin with but is partly open now. It looks pretty strange but okay. Since I don't have my new artificial eye yet, I have a temporary clear lens, so my eye looks completely red. Really Weird! But it is healing really well, and we can tell that when all the swelling and bruising is gone it will look as good as new.*

The next few days at the hotel consisted mainly of resting, ice packs, acetaminophen, and takeout. My new eye remained extremely swollen and bruised for several days. Eventually the swelling started to go down and the bruising changed from dark purple to light brown. In the morning, if my eyelids were stuck together, I would hold a warm facecloth on my eye for a few minutes until it would open naturally. The doctor told me it was important not to pry it open to avoid hurting my eyelids.

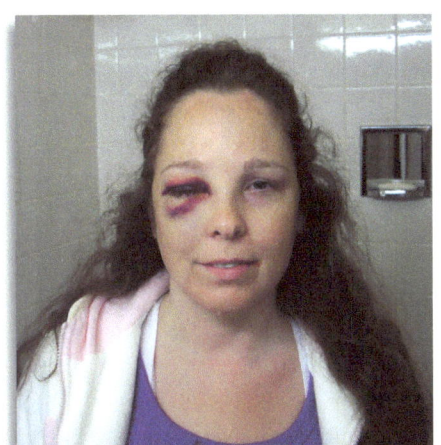
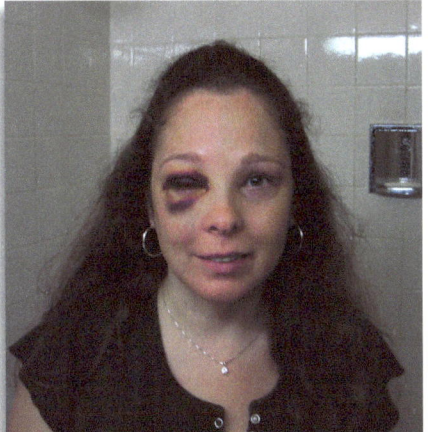
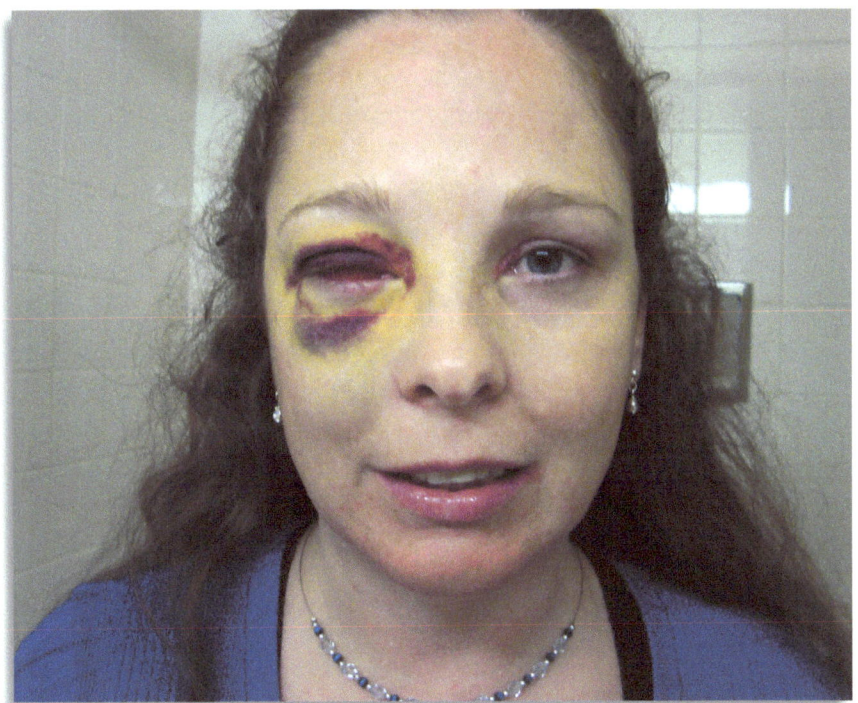

These pictures were taken on August 1-3, 2004.

Each afternoon once Gary was caught up on work, we would take a long walk on the streets surrounding our hotel. It was nice to be outside in the fresh air, moving around and taking in the sights. For safety, Gary held my hand on my blind side as occasionally I would forget about my missing depth perception and trip off curbs or forget to look to my right when crossing a street. As much as I loved the sunshine, since my surgery, bright lights and direct sunlight gave me an instant headache. I bought a pair of glaucoma sunglasses at a local pharmacy that fit over my regular eyeglasses. They were extremely helpful as they blocked out the light coming in from the top and sides of my glasses. They became my regular sunglasses for many years to come. After a few days, I felt well enough to add shopping to our daily activities; this greatly improved my mood. Once Gary and I thoroughly explored the mall, we checked out some of the stores located along the main streets. We enjoyed wandering around the little shops and picking out unique items to bring back home.

One evening we called Gary's mother, Muriel. We called Matt every day, but by this point we had been gone for over a week and wanted to update Muriel on my progress and get her opinion on how things were going back home. We were both feeling homesick, missing our son, our pets, and our comfortable home. Muriel said she had been stopping by the house every day to check on Matt and the pets and they were all doing fine. She was taking Jody for a walk every evening, and she was really enjoying it. She said if Jody got too excited and started pulling on the leash, she would say, "Slow down for Grammy," and Jody would slow right down for her. Our sweet Jody was such a gentle giant. Muriel said Kitty was doing fine as well. He would run out to greet her whenever she came over, demanding she pet him for a while. I was grateful to have Muriel and Matt back home looking after Jody and Kitty, but I was worried they were feeling abandoned and depressed.

The next day, we got up early to go to my final appointment with Dr. McGowan. I was feeling much better, but I didn't have time for my usual twenty minutes of icing, so I was feeling some pain and pressure. We walked down to the Princess Margaret Hospital and went up to the Ocular Oncology Clinic. I wore one of my colourful homemade eyepatches to match my outfit. When I was in public, I preferred wearing an eyepatch instead of a white gauze eye pad, otherwise people would stare and often ask questions. I was still feeling wounded and fragile, and I wasn't yet interested in relaying my situation to complete strangers, especially since most people looked horrified at the mere mention of eye cancer.

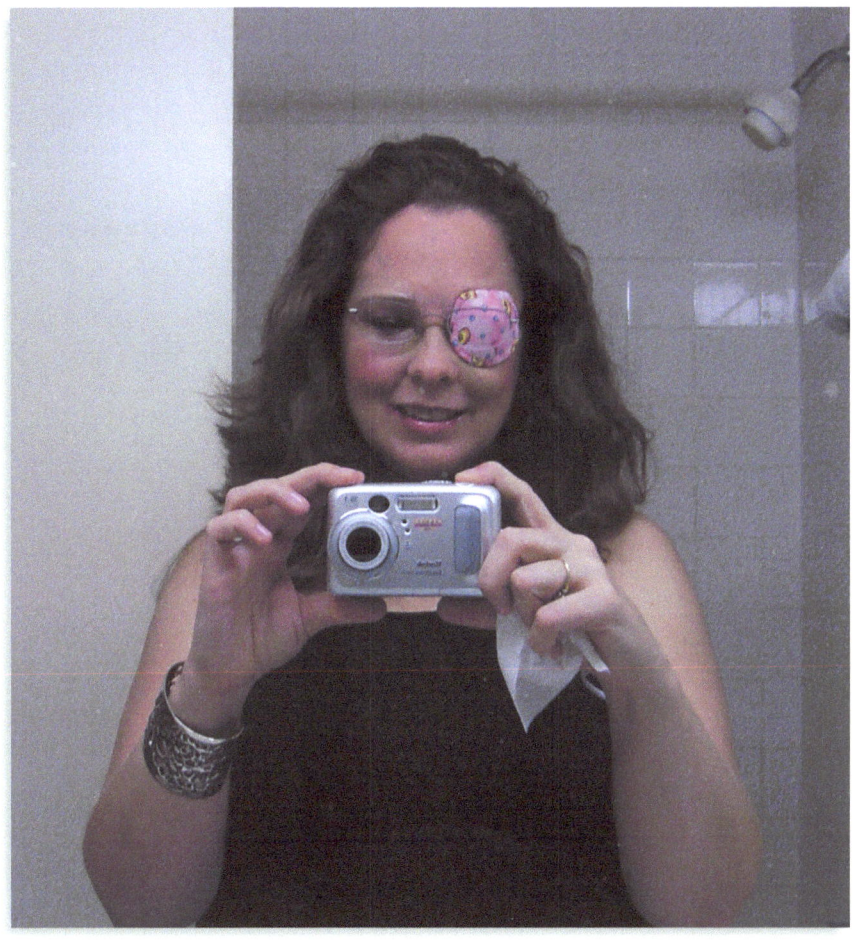

*I took this picture just before we left to go to my appointment.
I loved that my eyepatch covered the remaining swelling and bruising.
It felt good to fix my hair and put on make-up.
August 5, 2005.*

As we waited in the examination room, I thought about how much things had changed since the last time we were in the clinic and the doctors told me I had cancer. I had somehow accepted that my eye was gone, and I felt fortunate I would look and feel normal once I got a prosthetic eye. I was tired of the irritation and pain and hoped it would go away soon, but I was happy we would finally be going home to see Matt and our pets and sleep in our own bed.

When Dr. McGowan came into the examination room, he immediately complemented my eyepatch. I was happy he noticed it; I was hoping he would recognize my efforts to heal as quickly as possible and embrace my situation. I was determined to make him proud of my progress and not feel like his expertise was wasted on me. He examined me and said I was healing well and cleared me to travel home. He said I would need to heal for six more weeks before I could be fitted with a prosthetic eye. I also needed to have regular check-ups with a local ophthalmologist to closely monitor my remaining eye. The test results from my enucleated eye wouldn't be available for another couple of weeks; Dr. McGowan said he would call me at home with the results. Gary and I went back to the hotel, packed up all of our things, and checked out.

CHAPTER 12

SEEING THINGS DIFFERENTLY

Since Gary and I had gotten up earlier than usual to go to my final appointment, I was feeling tired and anxious. I was worried about the extremely long drive, but we both desperately wanted to go home; we made our way out of the city and toward the highway. After a couple of hours on the road, I started to cry. I was trying to be strong and tough it out, but I was in pain, feeling nauseated and stressed out. We pulled off the highway and stopped at a gas station where I took some medication, filled my ice pack, and got a few snacks. After our short break I started feeling better. Back in the car, I leaned my seat back, put my ice pack on my face, and we continued our journey.

Once we were on the open highway, I was looking at the scenery, and it became painfully obvious to me that there was a significant change in my vision. Despite it being a sunny summer day, it was as if there was a grey screen over everything. The bright beautiful world I remembered had become flat, grey, and dull. I told myself I would eventually adjust, and I was grateful to be alive, but it was still a sad realization.

I slept for the majority of the drive, waking periodically for washroom breaks, medication, and ice. By the time we arrived home, it was morning.

Matt, Jody, and Kitty were elated to see us. With the help of Muriel, Matt did a great job looking after the house and pets, and he even mowed the lawn. We were grateful for his help, and we were proud of how responsible he had become. He offered to help me in any way he could, but at that point I just needed to rest. I could hardly believe it was over. I was finally back home, and somehow I had to go back to my regular life without my eye.

As Gary and Matt unloaded the car, I ducked into the washroom. Looking at my face in the washroom mirror of my own house was a new level of realization. My bruised face and new red eye reminded me of my traumatic experience. It was still difficult to believe I had cancer and my eye was gone forever. I was sad, tired, and feeling a significant amount of pain and pressure in my temple and eye socket.

The following day, Matt went out with a friend and Gary went to check on things at his office while I attempted to unpack and organize things at home. At one point the phone rang. It was Dr. McGowan's receptionist calling to advise there would be a $700 charge for my implant. I was surprised by this information since it was the first time I was told about it. I decided to call Gary and let him know. As his phone started to ring, I realized I could hear it ringing in the house. He had left his phone at home by mistake and I would not be able to reach him. I suddenly panicked; I felt alone and afraid. The combination of being overtired, overwhelmed, and unsure about my future finally took its toll. As the tears started streaming down my face, I began to think about everything I had just been through and how my life had profoundly changed. I felt so disappointed that I had been surgically altered and I would never be whole again. I no longer felt independent or invincible, and I was worried Gary would eventually get tired of caring for me and leave.

Before long, Gary arrived home and found me curled up on the floor of our bedroom, sobbing. He did his best to comfort me, reassuring me the worst was over, and all I needed to do was rest and recover. He helped me take my anti-anxiety medication and then tucked me into bed where I slept for the next several hours with my sweet animals cuddling next to me.

CHAPTER 13

HEALING AT HOME

Over the next few days, I continued to use an ice pack, especially in the morning, as that was when the pain and swelling was at its worst. We all returned to our usual routines, and I started feeling much more like myself. I was still having a hard time getting used to my missing depth perception and would regularly hurt myself. I often hit my shoulders on door frames, regularly hit my head on just about anything, and made a great deal of mess trying to use the kitchen.

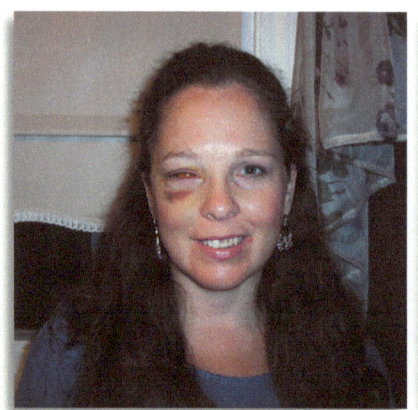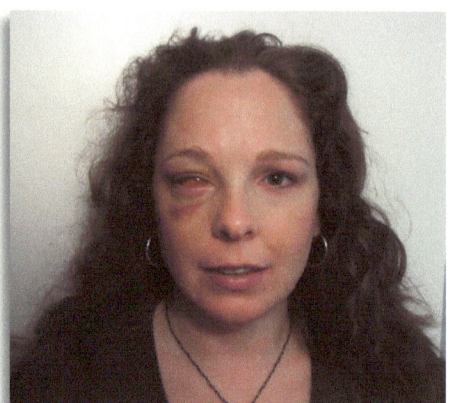

These pictures were taken during our first few days home from Toronto. August 6-8, 2004.

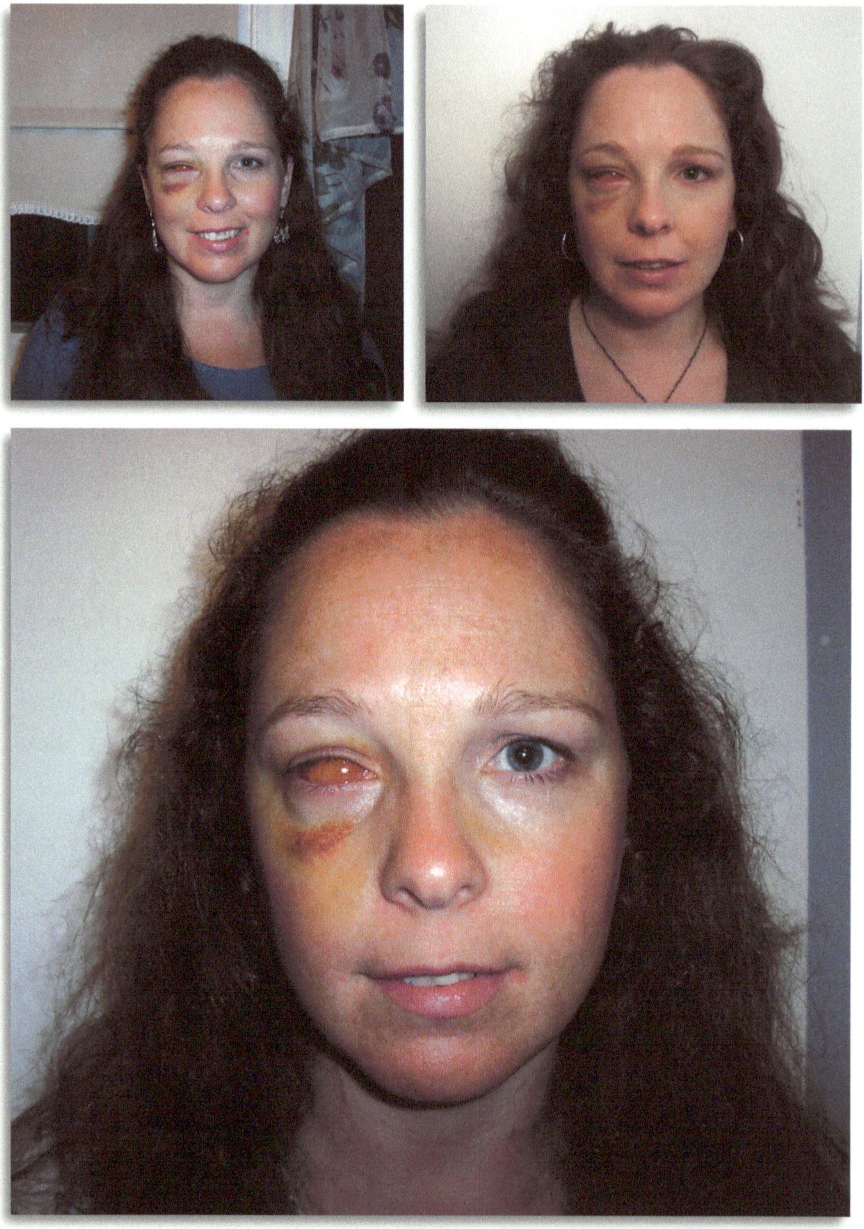

One evening while Matt was out with friends, Gary and I cuddled up together on the living room couch and watched a movie. We enjoyed having some much-needed quiet time together. When the movie was over, I walked into the kitchen to get a glass of water. I switched on the light, but I couldn't understand why it was so dark in the stairwell to my right. At first, I thought the light in the stairwell was burnt out but when I looked over, I saw the light was on and I realized, for a moment, I had forgotten about my missing eye. It was a strange sensation, but it made me feel hopeful I would eventually forget about my blind side altogether.

My new eye was feeling much better, although it was constantly watering and feeling itchy and sore and my head still had a great deal of pressure. It also seemed like my brain was still confused about my missing eye as I could still see white and black lines and shapes over everything. Prior to my surgery, I had thoroughly read all of the pamphlets I was provided and researched eye removal recovery and the possible complications online. I was fully aware of the pain, swelling, and bruising, but I did not read anything about my new eye watering and feeling irritated all of the time or the vision in my remaining eye being affected by white and black lines and shapes over everything. I was disappointed and extremely concerned that these issues were a permanent part of my new reality.

Ten days after surgery, the bruising was almost gone, and I no longer felt the need for an afternoon nap. I had a minimal amount of pain, however, I realized if I leaned forward, I would immediately get a headache and feel pain and pressure in my eye socket. Unfortunately, my new eye was still frequently watering, causing irritation and discomfort. Around this time, I noticed I was missing some of the sensation in my eyelids. If I touched my eyelids, I could feel it and they were working fine, but I couldn't tell if my new eye was open or closed without looking in the mirror. I realized that without an eyeball for my eyelids to work with, the sensation in my eyelids had changed.

I still wasn't ready to drive but, as often as possible, I would leave the house with Gary to run errands. Unfortunately, after shopping I would usually feel dizzy and nauseated but I couldn't figure out why. One day while we were at the grocery store, the cause of my dizziness revealed itself. Gary had left the aisle to pick up something and when he returned, he saw me spinning around like a ballerina holding a can of corn. I had no idea I was doing it, but I was spinning in an effort to see what was in my blind spot. With help from Gary, I stopped spinning and the nausea and dizziness went away.

By the two-week post-surgery mark, I started getting used to my field of vision, and I wasn't noticing the void as much. I also realized I wasn't hitting my head or shoulders as much. I was thankful for these small victories; however, I was starting to develop a new issue. Since the swelling was going down in my new eye, the acrylic conformer kept threatening to pop out. If I rubbed my eye, my bottom lid would go under the conformer and I would have to pull my bottom eyelid down to pop it back into place. I was worried the conformer would come out and I would lose it, or I wouldn't be able to put it back in.

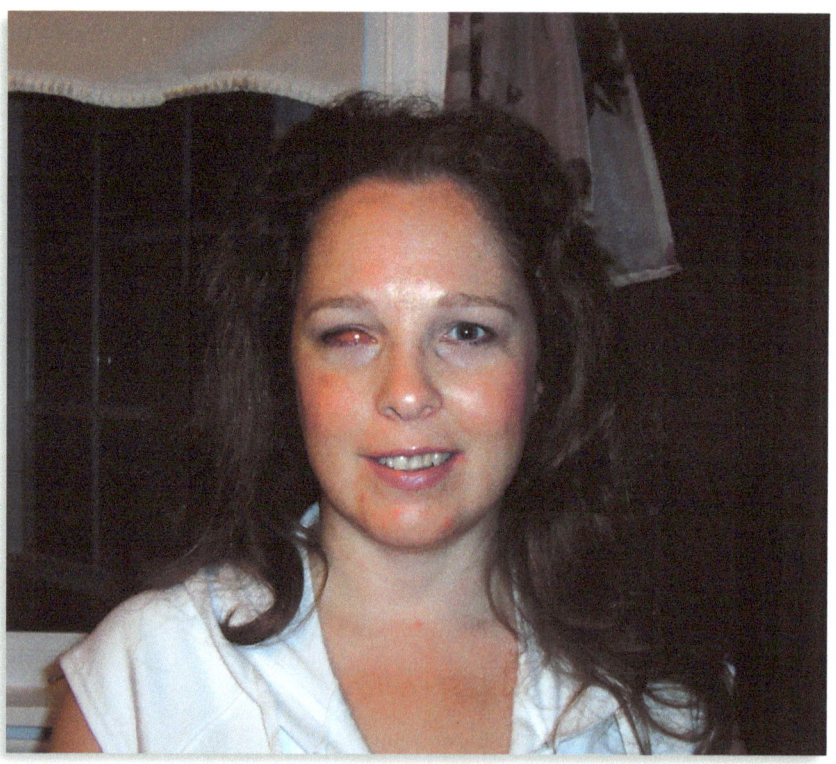

This picture was taken two weeks after my surgery.
August 12, 2004.

The following is the journal entry I wrote about how I was feeling at this time.

> *Friday August 13, 2004: Sometimes I look in the mirror and I'm still shocked that I lost my eye. It's such a blow. I mean I feel like I've been in an awful accident and something traumatic happened like someone died and I'm just beginning to deal with it.*

During this time, I would often go out and work in my garden. Being in the warm sunshine and working with my hands was therapeutic for me. Pulling weeds, pruning plants, and planting flowers helped me get used to my missing depth perception, and the peacefulness helped me come to terms with what I had gone through. It was rewarding to have a well-manicured garden and watch my beautiful flowers grow.

When I reached the three-week post-surgery mark, I contacted an ocularist and set up an appointment for September 15, 2004. I was told the prosthetic eye was not covered by Medicare and there would be an up-front cost of $1400. I was surprised to say the least. I contacted my employee medical insurance company and was relieved to find out they covered up to 80%. The hospital hadn't mentioned this cost and it wasn't in any of the pamphlets. Since I needed a letter from my surgeon for the insurance company, I called Dr. McGowan's office and asked about this hidden cost. I was told if I was a resident of Ontario, the majority of the cost, including my implant, would be covered by Medicare. I was thankful I had opted for a full medical insurance package through work. (New Brunswick now has an Ocular Prosthesis Program to help offset some of the costs, effective March 2018.)

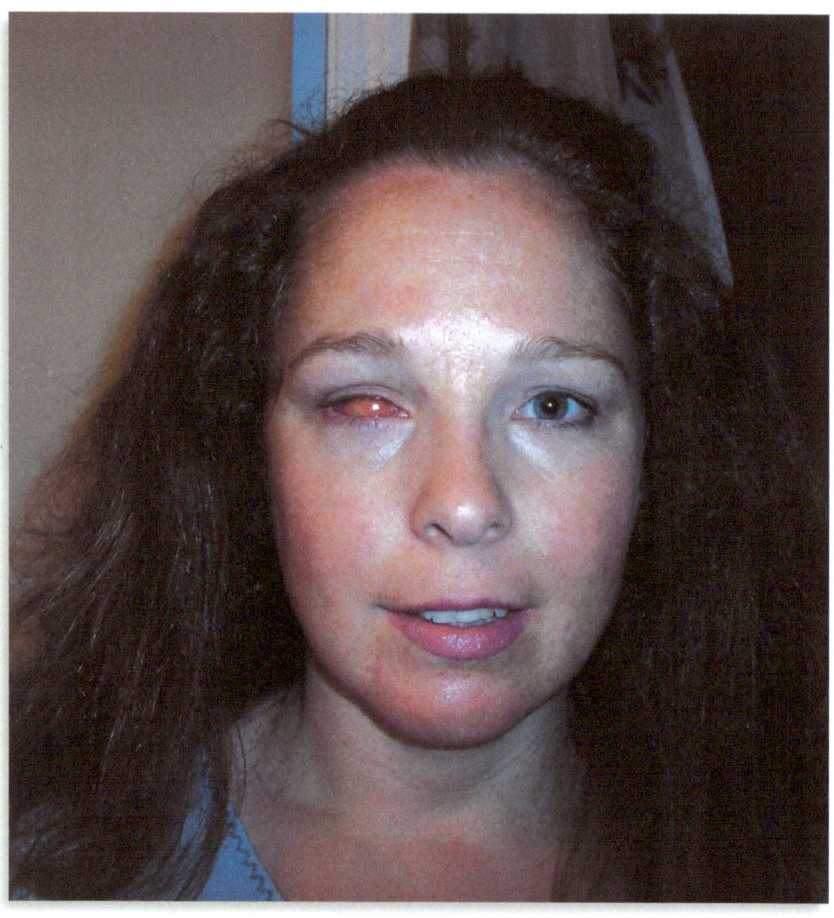

*This picture was taken three weeks after my surgery.
I was looking and feeling much more like myself.
August 19, 2004.*

Around this time, I also contacted my HR representative at work and advised her of my progress. I told her I wanted to wait until I had my prosthetic eye fitted before I returned to work. She understood and was completely accommodating. Even though my colleagues and managers were sympathetic to my situation, I was nervous about returning to work and feeling the need to recount my experience. I could barely talk about my surgery with my caring and supportive close friends and family members without immediately feeling flushed and having heart palpitations. I was still feeling fragile and traumatized from the shock of my diagnosis, the pain I experienced after surgery, and the disappointment of my new reality.

Near the end of August, I was feeling much better physically, but mentally I was still struggling. Most days would start off fine but eventually I would feel frustrated and angry. I was trying to move on with my life: work on my house, garden, and other projects, but my eye issues kept interfering. My new eye was feeling irritated and constantly watering. Since I was often wiping the tears away, the skin at the corners of my new eye had become raw and painful. I was also extremely disappointed with my vision. Without depth perception, everything looked dull and flat, and the issue with the lights and shadows was not going away either. Often, just looking in the mirror and seeing my red eye was enough to make me feel disappointed and frustrated. I tried to be grateful I was alive, but I was having a hard time.

The following is the journal entry I wrote describing the issue I was having with the lights and shadows.

> *Wednesday, August 18, 2004: The lights still aren't going away but I'm getting better at ignoring them and just focusing on what I do see. They are very distracting. It's kind of like having a bunch of geometrical shapes floating around. They are moving very slowly sort of like the spirograph screen saver on my computer. It makes me wonder if my vision will ever be clear again and, when my eyes are closed, if I'll ever see complete darkness again.*

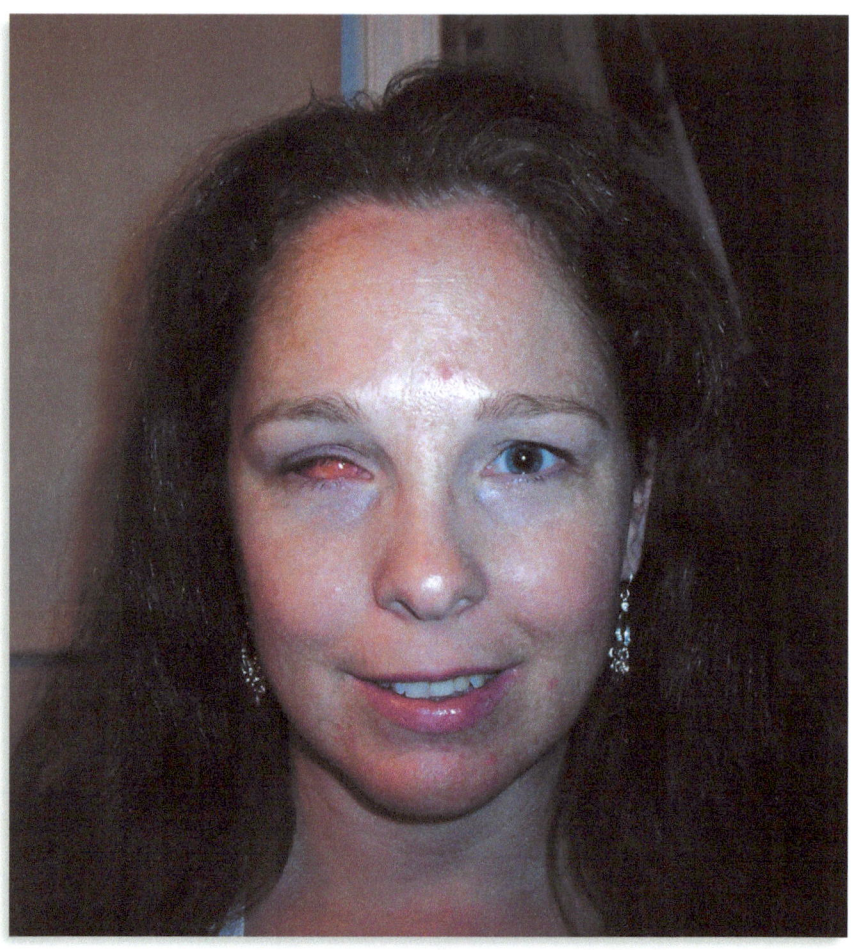

*By the end of August, other than my red eye,
I looked normal and felt ready for my prosthetic eye.
August 26, 2004.*

One evening, I was feeling defeated. I had hoped once we moved into our new house and Matt finished high school, our lives would become less complicated and more exciting. It felt like a dark cloud was following me around. Prior to my cancer diagnosis, I had been doing my best to live a healthy life: exercising, healthy eating, not smoking, and limiting alcohol. I had hoped all of my efforts would mean I would avoid getting cancer at a young age like my mother, but instead I was three years younger than her when I was diagnosed. I wondered what I had done wrong and if I continued to live my life in the same manner as I did before, would I end up getting cancer again? I was horrified knowing my body could make a deadly disease and, for all I knew, it could still be in my body wreaking havoc. I felt like a sitting duck and no matter what I did, it could come back with a vengeance and kill me. I talked to Gary about my fears. He was convinced I would be fine since the cancer was caught early. He told me I didn't do anything wrong and thought I was most likely genetically predisposed to get eye cancer. I appreciated his efforts, but I felt like I had wasted so much of my life. If I only had a few good years left, what was I going to do to make the most of it?

I wrote the following journal entry when the gravity of my situation finally hit me.

> *August 22, 2004. My life has drastically changed. Not so much in the physical area, but mentally and, well, I guess in the dreams and wishes I've had my whole life. I've always imagined being a singer or an actress or a dancer or a really great number of things that are unique and uncommon. Now it's different. When I think, "I could do that," I now wonder, "Could I?" I just don't know. It's kind of stupid because it's so unlikely that I would ever end up in any of the dream scenarios, but, well, this situation interferes with my fantasy. I no longer feel like I can do and be whatever I choose but now I'm faced with my reality. Reality bites! It's far too ordinary for my expectations [of] life ... Where do I go from here? How do I just pick up the pieces and go on? ... Not only is my eye gone and replaced with flashes of light and floating geometrical figures that drive me to distraction, but they had to use the C word! Don't give me that death sentence! I don't want to hear it! I haven't done anything yet! I have a whole life to live.*

After a rant like that, one would think I would've come up with a way to live my life more intentionally, however, I was still trying to recover and in no position to do anything profound. I tucked my feelings aside and continued with my regular day-to-day life hoping someday I would be well enough to follow my dreams.

Around this time, I decided to touch up the paint on some of the trim inside our house. I had been painting for most of my life, but this would be my first time painting since I lost my eye, and I was a little nervous. I climbed a few steps up the ladder and immediately felt dizzy. I considered getting down, but I was determined to continue; after a couple of minutes, the dizziness subsided. At first it was difficult to tell where I was putting my paint brush, so I tried looking at the brush from the side so I could compensate for my missing depth perception. After a few missteps and messes, I managed to figure it out and successfully completed painting the trim. I realized I might not be able to do things the same way I did before I lost my eye, but through trial and error, I would find a new way.

One evening, Gary and I went out to dinner at one of our favourite restaurants, and we started talking about our wedding. When we got engaged the previous summer, we had only planned to wait one year before we were married. We wanted to have an evening ceremony and reception in the backyard of our new house. We would string up lights, have multiple lanterns, bouquets of white roses, lots of food and music, and include all our friends and family. We were looking forward to getting married but since it had been such a difficult year, we decided to postpone our wedding until the following summer. By then I would be fully healed, and all the chaos would be behind us. I also knew I wouldn't have my prosthetic eye until the middle of September, and I really wanted it for our wedding photos. I was disappointed to wait, but I was also a little relieved since I wasn't ready to celebrate. I was still feeling fragile, beaten-down, and traumatized, and the idea of entertaining was overwhelming.

In early September, I spent the afternoon with one of my friends. It was the first time I had gone to a shopping mall without Gary since my surgery. It was really nice to catch up and discuss common interests with my old friend, but before long I had an accident. While we were chatting and walking through a department store, I ran into a stack of boxes, knocked them all down, and I nearly fell. The only thing I hurt was my pride, but

I certainly could've been seriously injured. The experience reminded me I was still getting used to the changes in my vision, and I needed to be much more careful.

A few days later, after a marathon of housework, I noticed some bloody discharge coming out of my new eye. It was concerning, but I assumed I had just been doing too much. When I woke up the next morning, my new eye was crusted over and glued shut. I used a warm cloth on my eye and cleaned it up, but then my eyelid would only open halfway. I was also feeling exhausted, had a headache, and I was feeling pressure in my chest. I was certain I was just overtired; I tried to take it easy for the rest of the day. That night I slept for eleven hours and woke up the following morning feeling much better.

On September 7, 2004, Dr. McGowan called with the test results from my enucleated eye. He said I had diffuse iris melanoma, which was worse than he had originally thought. Along with the tumour in my iris, the cancer was like spray paint with tiny particles scattered throughout my eye. Dr. McGowan was confident he was able to remove my eye without the cancer spreading, but he could not be 100% sure. I was relieved to hear I would not need to have chemotherapy or any other type of cancer treatment. He did, however, say I would have to have cancer screening tests every six months for the following five years to detect the cancer if it metastasized. I thanked him and hung up the phone with a pit in my stomach. At that moment, I realized my choice to delay surgery may have cost me my life.

CHAPTER 14

LOOKING NORMAL?

My ocularist appointment was only a week away. I was feeling excited about having two eyes again and looking normal. It was also the first step toward resuming my regular life, which included returning to work. As much as I enjoyed being home, I was feeling restless and bored, and I missed my friends.

On September 15, 2004, I met with an ocularist. The first thing he did was remove the acrylic conformer, which was painless as it popped right out. The next step was to make a mould by filling my eye cavity with liquid pink wax; this didn't really hurt but it felt rough under my eyelid. Taking the wax out was a little painful, but it only lasted a few seconds. He then made an acrylic copy of the shape using the new wax mould. Once completed, the ocularist hand-painted an iris and a pupil on the surface of the acrylic copy while looking at my good eye for reference. It was a fascinating process and required a great deal of precision. Unfortunately, I wouldn't be leaving with my new eye, as he needed to keep it overnight to harden.

The next day, I was excited I would finally have my new prosthetic eye, but my eyelid was red and painful, and my eye was watering. When we arrived at the ocularist's office, my prosthetic eye was put in place and I was handed a mirror. It was certainly nice to see two eyes on my face, but my new eye didn't look real. I thought it would look just like my old eye—perfect right away—but the prosthetic eye was much larger and looked lifeless. The ocularist tried to reassure me saying it would look better in a month or so once the swelling went down, but I couldn't help feeling disappointed. I tried to remain hopeful that it would look better in time, but I was feeling sad and overwhelmed. It certainly didn't help that my eye was feeling raw, swollen, and sore.

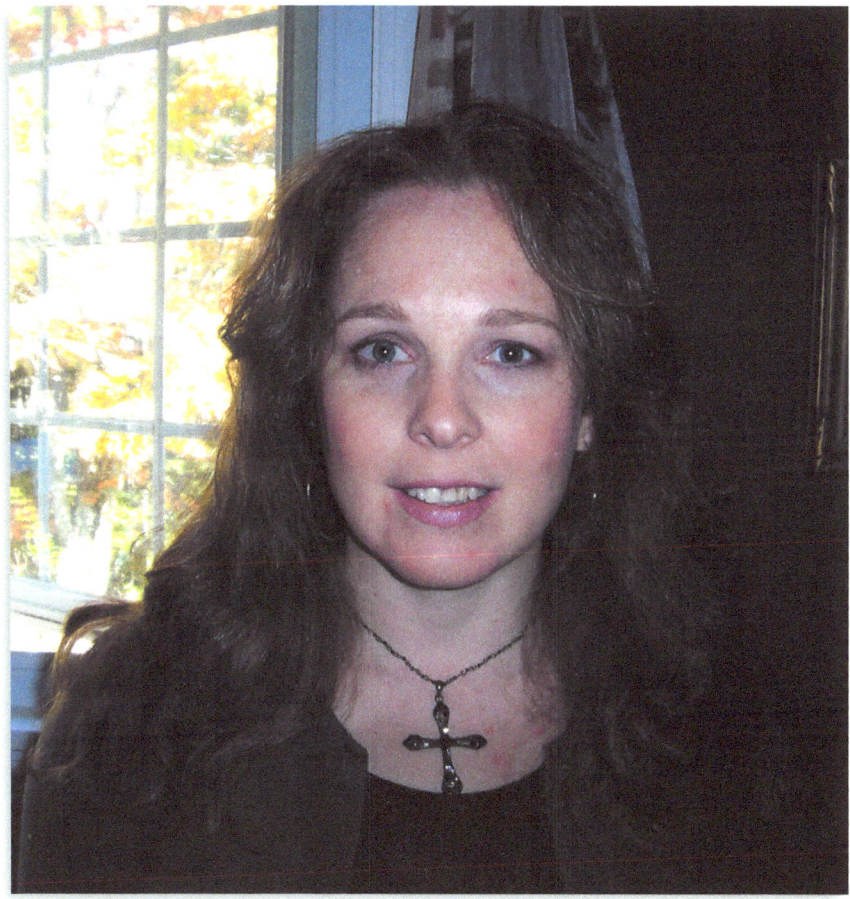

This picture was taken the day I was fitted with my new prosthetic eye. September 16, 2004.

The ocularist set up another appointment to see him in two months for my final fitting. He also gave me several pamphlets and some advice including how to remove my prosthetic eye, proper cleaning habits, and how to apply make-up to disguise the differences between my two eyes. I was thankful for the information, but I was surprised I needed to use make-up to disguise my new eye. Judging by the information and pamphlets I was given while we were at the Ocular Oncology Clinic in Toronto, I was under the impression my new prosthetic eye would look just like my real eye.

When I got home, I looked at my prosthetic eye again and could not believe how big it was and how little it moved. I couldn't help feeling defeated as I had hoped my new eye would make me feel normal again. I reminded myself what the ocularist said about the swelling, but I was losing hope. Dr. McGowan had mentioned the option of getting a motility peg in my implant to help the prosthetic eye move. He told me a titanium screw would be inserted into my implant and my prosthetic eye would have an indent in the back to fit the peg. This would enable my prosthetic eye to move almost as much as my real eye. I was not comfortable with the idea of having another procedure, and I was worried about the possible complications, but I knew it was an option if I was unhappy with the final result.

Over the next week, my new eye had discharge and pain. The ocularist recommended using some eye drops for comfort but after a week it was getting worse, so I made an appointment with my ophthalmologist, Dr. Purdy. He examined me and said I had formed pustules under my eyelid. He said it looked like I was having an allergic reaction to the acrylic conformer used after my surgery to shape my implant. He prescribed some antibiotic steroid eye drops (Tobradex-OP tobramycin/dexamethasone) to use four times per day. I really hoped it would work as my new eye was always irritated and I was feeling frustrated. I also asked him about the lights and shadows I had been seeing since my eye was removed. He said I had a condition called phantom eye syndrome. The optic nerve that served my missing eye was still sending messages to my brain; he didn't know if it would go away or not, but after a year or more I would get used to it and not notice it as much.

The following is the journal entry I wrote describing how I was feeling after getting my new artificial eye.

> *Tuesday, September 21, 2004: My eye is alright. The eyelid is still very itchy and swollen and red but at least I have very little discharge now and it's mainly clear so that must be a good sign. I've been pretty depressed these days, and I don't know if it's because I have an [eye] infection and I feel like I'm being shoved down again or if it's because I took one look at my artificial eye and went "It looks fake." I guess to be honest, I'm rather disappointed with the look of it. I thought it would move better and look a little more alive. Don't get me wrong, I think the workmanship is fabulous, it's just the technology I'm a bit disappointed with. I guess I just thought it would work better. I guess the truth is that it's a fake eye so it's going to look a bit fake.*

A few days later, my eyelids were still red and irritated, and I had a headache. My new eye did look a little better though, as my top eyelid was beginning to stretch over my prosthetic, and it looked more natural. My lower eyelid didn't look right yet, as there was still too much white showing under the painted-on iris; I was hopeful this would also improve over time.

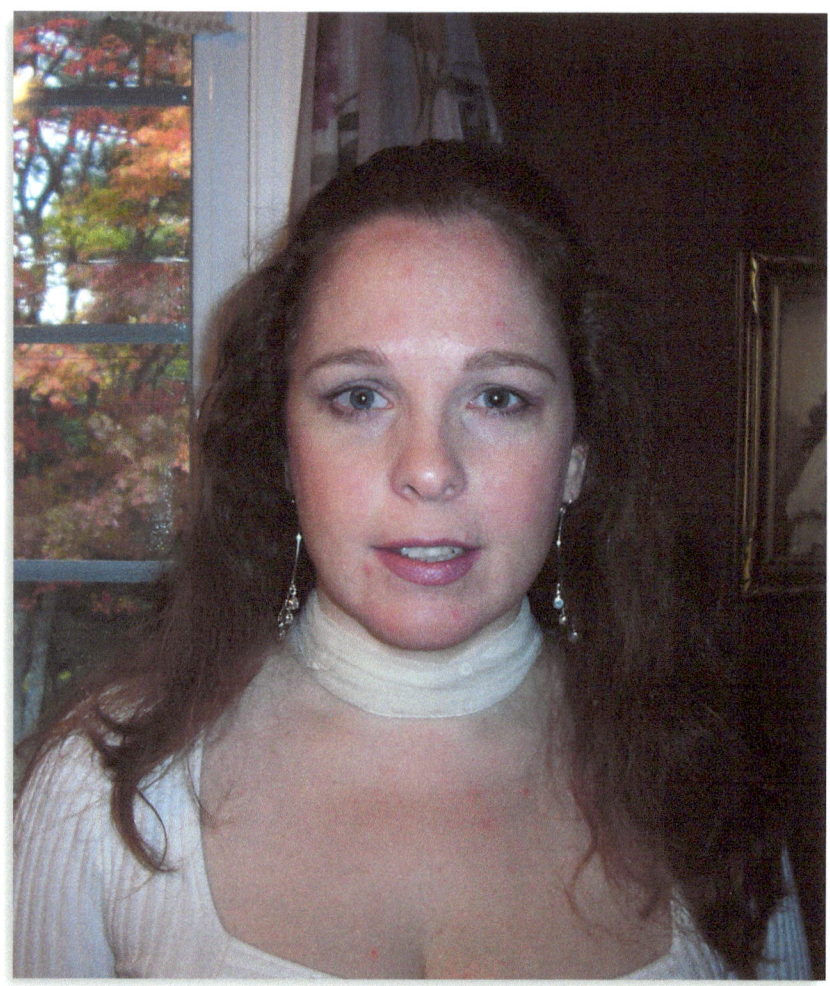

This picture was taken one week after I was fitted with my new prosthetic eye. September 23, 2004.

"Did you make a list?" Gary called from the kitchen one evening around 7:00 p.m. I was in the bedroom trying to decide what to wear; I was feeling puffy as I still hadn't lost the few pounds I had gained after my surgery. Gary and I were going to the grocery store to pick up a few supplies.

"It's on the counter," I told him.

I settled on a loose-fitting black cotton T-shirt and a pair of faded blue jeans and walked out to the kitchen. I checked over the list, put on my shoes and my jacket, and we left. When we arrived at the store, we walked hand in hand through the parking lot; Gary was still protective of me, especially around cars. We walked through the grocery store, picked up the items we needed and, while we were in the checkout line, my new eye started watering. I wiped away the tears from the corner of my eye and was suddenly worried I had made my prosthetic eye twirl. Over the past few days, Gary had noticed my eye was often pointing in the wrong direction, likely due to the swelling going down. It looked really strange because my iris and pupil would be in the top outer corner of my eye and barely visible. I walked over to a nearby window; it acted like a mirror since it was dark outside. I could tell by my reflection that my pupil was pointed to the top right. I felt panicked and immediately used my finger to move the prosthetic into the right position before anyone noticed. That's when I heard voices and realized there were people on the other side of the window watching me. I looked at their faces and I could see they were staring at me in shock. I was completely embarrassed and quickly moved away from the window and back to Gary. I told him about the people on the other side of the window and he just laughed and told me not to worry about it. I realized he was right, I had to accept the fact that I had an artificial eye and sometimes people would notice. After that, I no longer panicked if I thought my eye had twirled but I made sure to have a compact mirror with me at all times just in case it happened again.

Around this time, I decided to refinish our wooden kitchen chairs. I took them out to the garage and sanded them down, getting them ready for the new stain. When I was finished sanding, my eye was irritated and watering. I took out my prosthetic eye to clean it and inspect my implant. I could see a space had formed all the way around my implant, making room for my prosthetic eye to move. I rinsed off my prosthetic eye, put in some eye drops, and it felt much better.

I finally felt like I was beginning to adjust to single-eye vision. While walking Jody, if I turned my head slightly to the right, I could balance my view and almost eliminate my blind spot. This revelation was helpful a week later when I tried driving for the first time. I was nervous but Gary was patient and encouraging. To my surprise, my lack of depth perception was not an issue. I took my time and kept several car lengths between my car and the other cars, and everything turned out fine. I was also learning to live with phantom eye syndrome. I realized certain conditions made it worse, such as trying to see in the dark or bright lights. To offset these issues, we installed some dimmer switches and a few night lights.

A few days before my thirty-seventh birthday I was feeling depressed. I was reflecting on what I had gone through over the past year, and I was still feeling traumatized. I was unhappy I hadn't lost the extra weight I'd gained, and I still hadn't started back to work so I was feeling restless and bored. I wasn't even sure I wanted to go back to my old job. I wondered if I should consider going back to school or changing careers. Before I got cancer, I felt like I had plenty of time to do whatever I wanted with my life and the next exciting adventure was just around the corner. Being diagnosed with cancer gave me a reality check, and I was afraid I would run out of time before I got a chance to experience some of the great things life had to offer.

When my birthday arrived, I woke up early and made some breakfast. As I sipped my coffee, I thought about my birthdays when Matt was young. Since I always brought him breakfast in bed on his birthday, he would insist on bringing me breakfast in bed. It usually involved copious amounts of sugar and me trying to choke it down so I wouldn't disappoint him. I fondly remembered his birthday when he turned seven years old with his shaggy blond hair, big blue eyes and infectious smile. That year he woke up before me, so I asked him if he still wanted to have breakfast in bed. He raced into his bedroom, jumped on his bed and waited for me to get his breakfast tray ready, all the while excitedly chattering to me from his room. He knew I had planned a special birthday breakfast with sugar cereal – a rare find in our house – and I also had a few small toys and a couple of treats for dessert. While he ate, I sat with him and we talked about all the fun things we were going to do on his special day. I didn't have a lot of money, but he was excited about the little things like spending five dollars at the dollar store, going to the park, and having fast food for dinner - another rare treat. He was so easy to please and seeing him happy brought me a great deal of joy. He wasn't much of a morning person anymore, so he was no longer interested in having or giving breakfast in bed, but I still made sure to pick up some special breakfast treats for him to have on his birthday every year. Later that day, Gary and Matt gave me a bouquet of pink and white roses and a few gifts, and in the evening, Gary took me out for a romantic dinner. I was grateful to have two wonderful men in my life making me feel special and loved.

Around this time, I watched *The Brooke Ellison Story*, a true story about a girl who was hit by a car and became a quadriplegic at eleven years old. Despite her limitations, Brooke went on to finish high school with honours, graduated magna cum laude from Harvard, and completed a master's degree. Her story put things into perspective for me. Many people like Brooke who were facing much greater obstacles than I was were accomplishing great things. Until that point, I felt like a cancer victim— broken and limited. Brooke's story made me realize my missing eye wasn't limiting me, it was my own perspective. After what I went through, it would have been understandable if I didn't go back to work, or if I became bitter, depressed, or withdrawn, but that wasn't me. I had always been a fighter, and I knew I could come back from this. I suddenly felt the need to get up, dust myself off, and be better and stronger than ever. Instead of focusing on what I had lost and my disadvantage, I started focusing on everything I had to be grateful for and started looking forward to the great things I was going to do with my life. I realized that whether I had a long life to live or not, I wanted it to be full and exciting. Unfortunately, my forward momentum hit a snag; I caught a horrible flu and was sick for the next few weeks.

As an infant I had been gravely ill with pyloric stenosis, a rare condition that blocks food from entering the small intestine and at three months old, I had corrective surgery (pyloromyotomy). Throughout my childhood, I continued to have stomach issues and was plagued with a variety of chronic infections. This caused my mother to be on high alert every time I started feeling sick. She would bring my pillow and blanket into the living room along with a colouring book, crayons, and a few of my favourite dolls, and put on some cartoons to help me pass the time. She was very attentive and would check on me often, taking my temperature and making my favourite meals and snacks. My mother had decided not to go back to work until after I started school; I was fortunate to have her close by during my young years. When I was well, we would run errands - usually to the grocery store or the bank, or we would visit neighbours and friends for tea and cookies. I would also help her with the housework and the cooking and baking. When it was time for me to go to school, my mother enrolled in secretary school. Each morning I admired how fancy she looked in one of her brightly coloured minidresses with matching silk scarf and high heel shoes. My mother had a beautiful hourglass figure, like one of my barbie dolls, and all of her clothing looked amazing on her. If there was time, she would let me help her pick out her jewelry; she always made me feel like we were a team and my opinion mattered. When I was a little older, she told me she would've loved to have been a nurse, but the course was much more expensive and took much longer than the secretary course and she couldn't afford it. I tried to encourage her to go back to school but she said it was too late for her and she was fine with being a secretary.

On November 9, 2004, for the first time in nearly six months, I went back to work. As I went up the elevator, I felt my heart pounding hard in my chest. I kept saying to myself, *You can do this, you can do this*, but I was feeling incredibly anxious as I walked through the office doors. I said hello to some of my co-workers as I went to meet my manager, who was expecting me. He advised me to go through my email and catch up on the latest procedural changes. As I sat at my desk, the familiar people and surroundings helped me feel comfortable, and I began to calm down. Countless friends and co-workers briefly stopped by to say hello and welcome me back. Eventually, I had a meeting with my manager and a return-to-work coordinator to discuss a plan to help me ease back into work. They were both extremely accommodating, and we agreed on four hours per day for three days each week.

After my meeting, I sat with one of my co-workers to watch her work for a while. Multiple times throughout the day, I found myself on the verge of tears; a feeling of sadness would wash over me, and I had to take some deep breaths to calm myself down. I was also feeling nervous and lost without Gary; a strange sensation since I had always been fiercely independent. By the time my shift was over, I was feeling overwhelmed and more than ready to leave. I left the office and found Gary waiting for me in the building's parking lot. I got into the front seat of the car and he said, "How did it go?" I immediately started crying. Through my tears I explained that everything went fine and it was really nice to see everyone, but it was extremely overwhelming. I felt silly for crying, but I didn't feel as strong as I used to be. I felt traumatized and wished I could erase the past six months from my memory and move on. I felt completely out of control of my emotions. I was sure I would feel better in time, but all I could think about while I was in the office was running out and never going back.

I tried to adhere to the return to work schedule we agreed upon, but I quickly discovered that after being in the office for less than an hour I would get a severe headache or a migraine. I consulted my ophthalmologist, and he recommended I use an anti-glare screen on my computer, avoid fluorescent lights, and have my eyeglasses modified to add a tint and an anti-glare treatment. He also recommended I slowly transition back to work to avoid too much eye strain.

Unfortunately, even with the recommended adjustments, I was still struggling with constant headaches. My eyesight in my remaining eye had diminished since I lost my eye, and I realized I was straining to see the small font on my work computer screen. Gary did some research and found a magnifier program called ZoomText. This program enlarged everything on my computer screen, making it much easier on my remaining eye. It would take several months, but with the special accommodations, I successfully returned to work full time.

In the middle of November, I had my final prosthetic eye fitting. After some small adjustments, my prosthetic eye fit the space much better and no longer twirled around or threatened to come out. It also looked much more like my other eye. For the first time in months, I felt normal and was happy with how I looked. My eye bothered me again for a while after the adjustment—it felt raw and it was watering—but after a week of eyedrops and rest, it settled down.

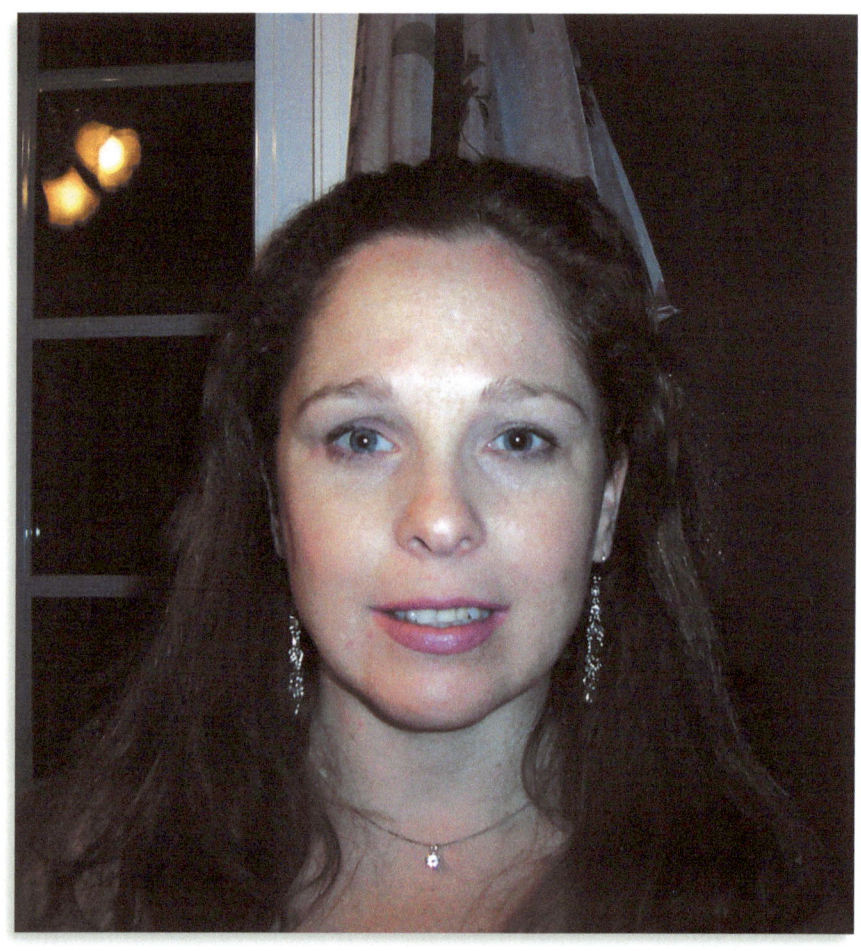

This picture was taken after I got home from my final fitting. My prosthetic eye is looking and feeling much better. November 18, 2004.

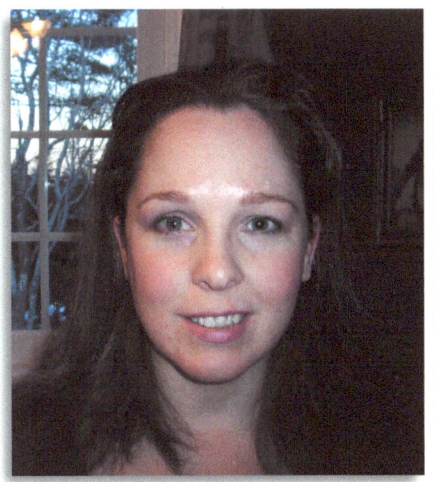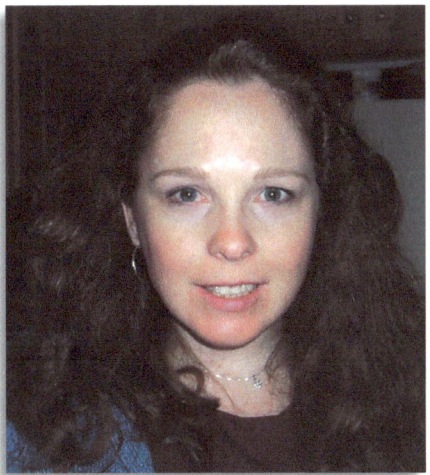

One week later it looked even better. I've also included my original photo with my two real eyes for comparison. Just a slight difference at this point. November 25, 2004.

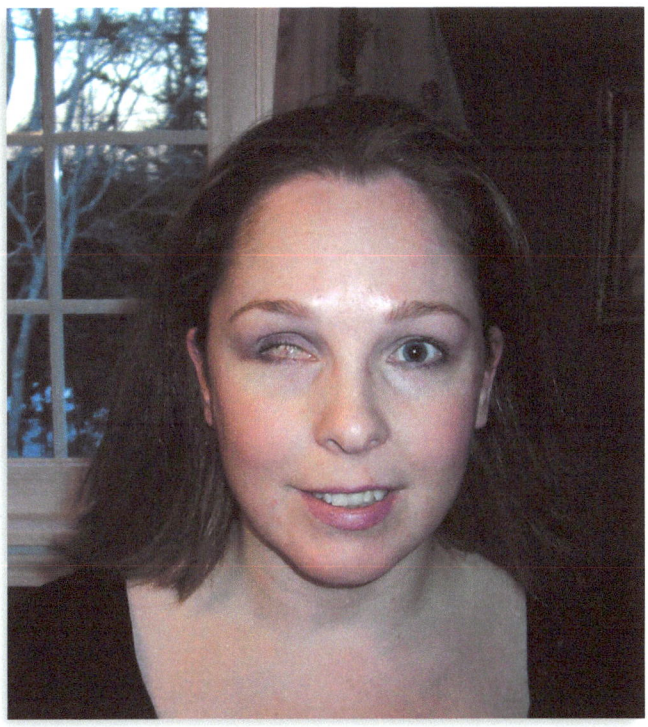

I removed my prosthetic eye to show the tissue covering my implant. It turned from red to pink and looked more like skin. November 25, 2004.

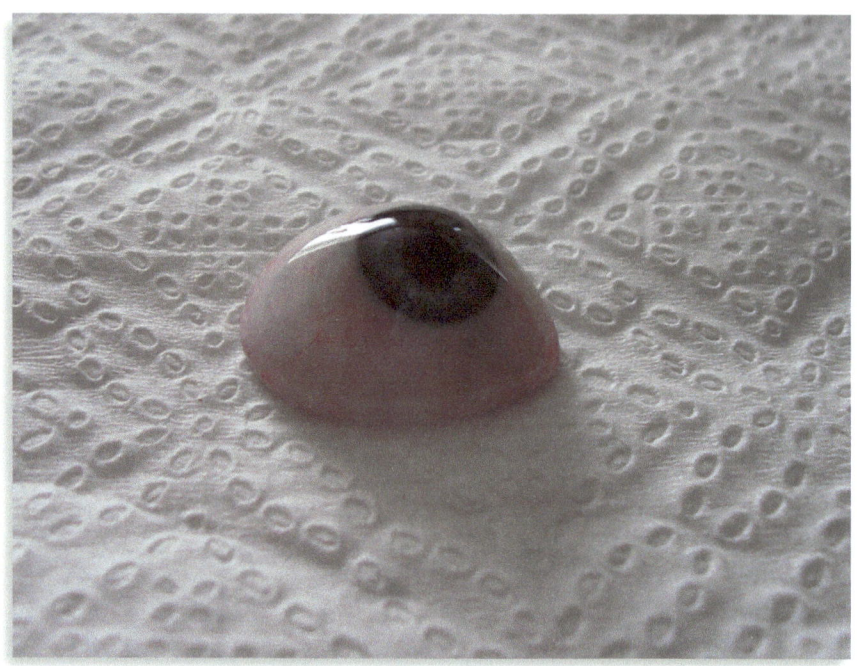

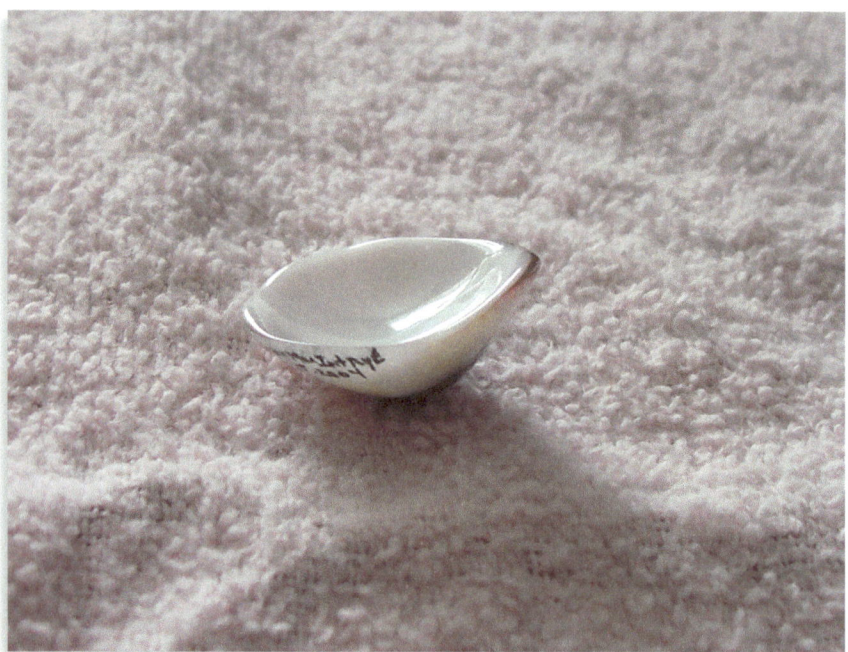

*The front and back of my prosthetic eye.
November 25, 2004.*

CHAPTER 15

CANCER SCREENING

In early December of 2004, I went to see my family doctor to have the tests ordered for my six-month post-surgery cancer screening. Knowing it would take a month or two for the tests to be scheduled, I wanted to get the process started. My doctor ordered a blood test and an ultrasound of my internal organs. With the tests ordered, I was able to focus my energy on getting ready for Christmas.

A few days before Christmas, I was feeling brave and decided it was time for a solo drive to the mall. I felt a little panicked at first, but I took some deep breaths, and I was fine. I took my time and stayed focused on everything and everyone around me. I parked as far away from the other cars as possible in a space I knew I could easily leave. I walked through the mall, picked up a few last-minute gifts, and made my way back home. After my outing, I knew I would still be able to drive. I would have to be careful, but it would be worth it to have my independence and the privilege of driving again. I felt liberated, and I was proud of myself for taking the first step.

Gary, Matt, and I had a wonderful Christmas; we spent some quality time together and with our extended family and friends. On Christmas Eve, we followed our usual tradition: we opened presents and then ate nachos, with my famous cream cheese dip, while watched a movie. We laughed together and had a great evening; it felt like we had returned to our pre-cancer lives.

Even though I tried my best to stay in the moment, thoughts of my upcoming medical tests would often cross my mind and cause a wave of anxiety to wash over me. I had faith in Dr. McGowan's expertise and his ability to contain the cancer, but there was a chance it could've gotten out. Knowing how dangerous my cancer was, I couldn't help wondering if this would be my last Christmas.

On December 31, 2004, I went to the hospital for an abdominal ultrasound. After I checked in, I was taken into a small, dark room with a bed and a computer, and I was asked to lie down. The technician put cold jelly on my bare stomach, and then she pressed a wand against it in several different areas. She scanned my liver, gallbladder, spleen, pancreas, and kidneys; the test took around thirty minutes. My follow-up doctor's appointment wasn't for a few weeks, so I tried to go on with my regular routine and avoid thinking about my test results.

During this time, I continued to have issues with my eye: irritation, discharge, headaches, and phantom eye syndrome. It had been almost six months since my surgery, and I was disappointed I was still dealing with these issues. I had come to terms with losing my eye, but these additional issues were hard to accept. I realized I would have to somehow find a way to accept my situation or I would become angry and bitter.

Adjusting to my lack of depth perception was certainly improving but I would still occasionally walk into things and have spills and messes. I started finding some new safeguards by using my other senses. I would listen for the sound of a door or drawer closing, or I would feel for the edge of a table or the counter before setting down a dish. Most of my accidents happened when I was in a hurry or the house was disorganized. I learned to be more organized by ensuring everything was in its place and by following through with housework and tidying up every evening before bed. I also gave myself more time to get ready before work to avoid the last-minute rush, otherwise I would feel stressed and anxious before I even left the house. These changes made my day-to-day life much less frustrating and, as a result, greatly improved my mood.

I was doing laundry the afternoon of January 10, 2005, when the phone rang. I put down the overflowing basket of towels and picked it up. The woman on the other end said she was calling from the hospital and wanted me to come in the following week for an abdominal CT scan. I asked her why, and she told me the paperwork indicated they would be looking at my liver, but she did not have any additional information and I should contact my doctor if I wanted to know more. My knees almost buckled, and I couldn't catch my breath. The doctors had told me if the cancer reached my liver, I would not survive. I knew there was a small chance the cancer could have gotten out of my eye, but six months had passed, and I had been feeling safe since I didn't have any unusual symptoms. I hung up the phone and went downstairs to Gary's office as the tears started to roll down my face. I was thankful Gary had decided to work from home that day as he was able console me. He told me I shouldn't jump to the worst conclusion as it was possible I was fine and it was a mistake or nothing serious.

The following is the journal entry I wrote that evening.

> *January 10, 2005: The hospital called and they want me to go in for a CT scan of my liver next week. I was pretty surprised. Dr. McKim never mentioned it so it made me think there may be something wrong on my last test. I got a little upset but then I realized there is no point. Even if they did see something it doesn't mean anything. I'm just going to have to get used to tests and re-tests.*

The following is the journal entry I wrote the next day.

> *January 11, 2005: I called the doctor's office today and they told me that the radiologist recommended a CT scan of my liver after he saw my ultrasound! So, I don't know what that means but I guess it doesn't matter right now. It's just a test and that's how I should look at it. I can't imagine what it*

would be like to head down the road of secondary cancer. Well, hopefully I'll be okay.

Despite my mother's life-altering mastectomy and debilitating cancer treatments, the cancer metastasized to her liver five years later, and she was diagnosed with terminal cancer. Before the cancer had returned, my mother was adjusting to life following her recent separation; after twenty-five years of marriage and countless hours of counselling, my parents had decided to go their separate ways. She had also been diagnosed with bipolar disorder (at the time it was called manic depression) and prescribed some medication that leveled out her mood swings and made her much happier. She was still working full time, but she spent as much time as possible with Matt and I. She adored her grandson and did everything she could for him. Matt loved his grandmother and would light up whenever she came to visit. When she walked through the door of our apartment, he would grab her hand and lead her to his favourite book or toy so she could play with him or read to him. My mother loved his attention and would always indulge him just to make him happy. I loved spending time with her too. I confided in her about everything happening in my life, often calling her multiple times each day; as a young single mother, I greatly appreciated her insight and advice. Since Matt's birth father and his family were not involved and provided no support financially or otherwise, my mother did her best to fill the gap. She regularly took us shopping, to the park or to various appointments. She also occasionally babysat in the evenings while I attended a night course as I had finally started going to university hoping to carve out a better life for Matt and I.

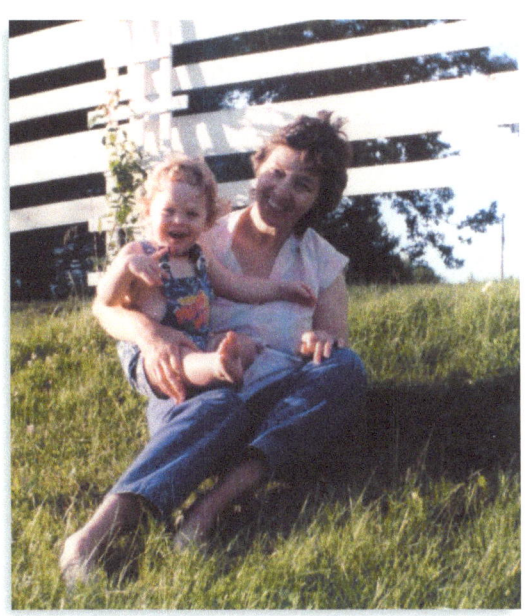

*My dear mother, Jeanette MacIntyre, with baby Matt.
She deeply loved her grandson and it broke her heart to leave him.
June 1987.*

At twenty-two years old, I had to say goodbye to my mother forever. Somehow, I had to find a way to go on and raise my little boy without her love and support. One day, I was in tears sitting at her bedside in the palliative care unit of the hospital when she put her hand on top of mine, looked into my eyes and said, "Sometimes bad things happen and it's not your fault. They just happen. Remember that you are a good girl and I will always love you." She then added, "You have a choice to either be angry or to rise above it." I appreciated her words of wisdom, but it would take years before I could put them into practice. Within two short months, I watched my beautiful, vibrant mother completely deteriorate, slip into a coma, and die. She was only forty-four years old. For years afterwards, I was haunted by reoccurring nightmares in which I was frantically searching for my sick or hurt mother. Each time I had one of these nightmares, I would wake up in tears and in a state of panic. Without my mother, my life changed significantly. My father remarried and was focused on raising his new family and, before long, they moved to Ontario. With very little support from family or friends, Matt and I were essentially on our own.

It broke my heart to think about leaving my fiancé and son. Gary and I were supposed to be planning our wedding and our future, not worrying about my demise. I knew Gary would look after Matt if anything happened to me, but I desperately wanted to be around to love and support him throughout his life in a way my mother couldn't be for me. As a young adult, the loneliness I felt from my mother's absence was difficult to deal with, and I frequently suffered from bouts of depression, panic attacks, and thoughts of suicide. Some days it was difficult to get out of bed, and other days I was paralyzed by fear and the thought of some other tragic event happening. It was no way to live or raise a child. Fortunately, through counselling and medication, I was able to eventually come to a place of acceptance, and I learned how to live without my mother.

Over the next few days, I did everything possible to distract myself from my upcoming test. I cleaned the house, organized some closets, and spent some quality time with Kitty and Jody. One afternoon, Jody and I went for a walk around our neighbourhood. The sun was shining but it was a cold and windy winter day. As we rounded a corner, a gust of cold air blew in my face and I immediately had what felt like an ice cream headache. I vaguely recalled being told my prosthetic eye would not be as protective as a real eye. I pulled my winter hat over my prosthetic eye and it provided some relief. The next time I went out in the cold, I wore a heavy eyepatch to protect my eye and the issue was resolved.

The day before my CT scan, I went to the hospital and picked up the CT scan dye. I had to mix the dye with cranberry juice, drink a portion the night before the test and drink the rest the day of the test. It tasted horrible! Knowing how bad it was, I set aside some extra time in the morning to get it down. I would later find out mixing the dye with lemon iced tea was a much better combination and not so difficult to drink.

On January 19, 2005, I woke up early and got ready to go to the hospital for my CT scan. This included choking down the rest of the cranberry juice and dye. When I was checking into the hospital, the admissions representative asked me for my next of kin. I advised her it was my fiancé, Gary. She told me I could only use Gary if we were married, otherwise

I would have to use a blood relative who was of legal age. This was news to Gary and I as the hospitals in Ontario did not have a problem naming Gary as my next of kin (this has since been changed in New Brunswick to include common law spouses). Gary was shocked by this news and said it was time for us to get married.

I wasn't sure if he was serious or not, but I didn't have time to talk to him about it then. We walked down to the waiting room, Gary took a seat, and a nurse led me to a back room to change into a hospital gown. Afterwards, the nurse told me she would be putting an IV in my hand as more dye needed to be injected during the test. I was not happy about the IV, but I needed to know what was going on with my liver. Fortunately, it was a small needle and she was able to get it in on the first try. The nurse brought me into a large room with a narrow bed sticking out of a giant white metallic circle. I was asked to lie on the bed and then she walked away, leaving me alone in the room. The bed moved in and out of the giant circle while a voice over a speaker told me to hold my breath occasionally for a few seconds. The scan took forty-five minutes. When the test was over, the nurse removed my IV, and told me I could get dressed and leave. Gary and I left the hospital hoping for the best. We would have to wait another week before we would find out the results at my upcoming doctor's appointment.

CHAPTER 16

WEDDING BELLS

That evening, while we were having dinner, Gary told me he was serious and wanted to get married immediately. He suggested having a civil ceremony as soon as possible and having a big reception at a later date. It wouldn't be my ideal summer garden wedding, but I agreed, and I was happy I was about to marry the love of my life. The next day, Gary contacted the courthouse. He found out there were quite a few dates available to book our ceremony, therefore, we would be able to get married as soon as we were ready. We immediately registered for a marriage license and ordered our wedding bands. It would take ten days for the wedding bands to be sized; with that in mind, we booked an appointment to have a Justice of the Peace marry us at the courthouse.

I was happy we were finally getting married, but I was nervous about my looming test results. I did my best to enjoy the planning phase and not let my fears put a damper on this happy time. It didn't help that I wasn't feeling well; I had constant pain and bloating in my stomach, and I was feeling nauseated and dizzy. I was hoping it was from the dye used for the CT scan and not from a cancerous tumour growing in my liver.

On January 27, 2005, Gary and I went to see my family doctor, Dr. McKim, for the results of my CT scan. Gary held my hand while we sat in the small examination room bracing ourselves for the news. The doctor came in, looked at the report and said I had a growth on my liver. He said they could not be 100% sure but the size and shape was consistent with a cavernous hemangioma. Dr. McKim explained further, telling us it was a benign tumour made up of a tangle of blood vessels. He said these types of tumours were rarely life-threatening or problematic, and my upcoming blood test would rule out any other abnormalities or concerns. We were elated. Hearing the word "benign" was a great relief to both of us.

Over the next couple of weeks, Gary and I were busy preparing for our wedding. We had originally planned to have a small, private ceremony, but since our friends and family members wanted to celebrate with us, we decided to make the arrangements to have a reception at our house following our wedding. We also decided to start the process for Gary to become Matt's legal guardian and to legally change Matt's last name. After a great deal of shopping, a few lawyer visits, and a couple of visits to a few government offices, we were finally ready to get married.

At 3:00 p.m. on February 18, 2005, I married the love of my life and best friend, Gary Nightingale. It was incredible to be standing in front of our closest family and friends committing ourselves to each other. Immediately following our wedding ceremony, Gary made the announcement that he had become Matt's legal father and Matt's last name had been changed to Nightingale. I was extremely grateful to Gary for taking the necessary steps to make this happen. Matt was excited and proud to officially be Gary's son.

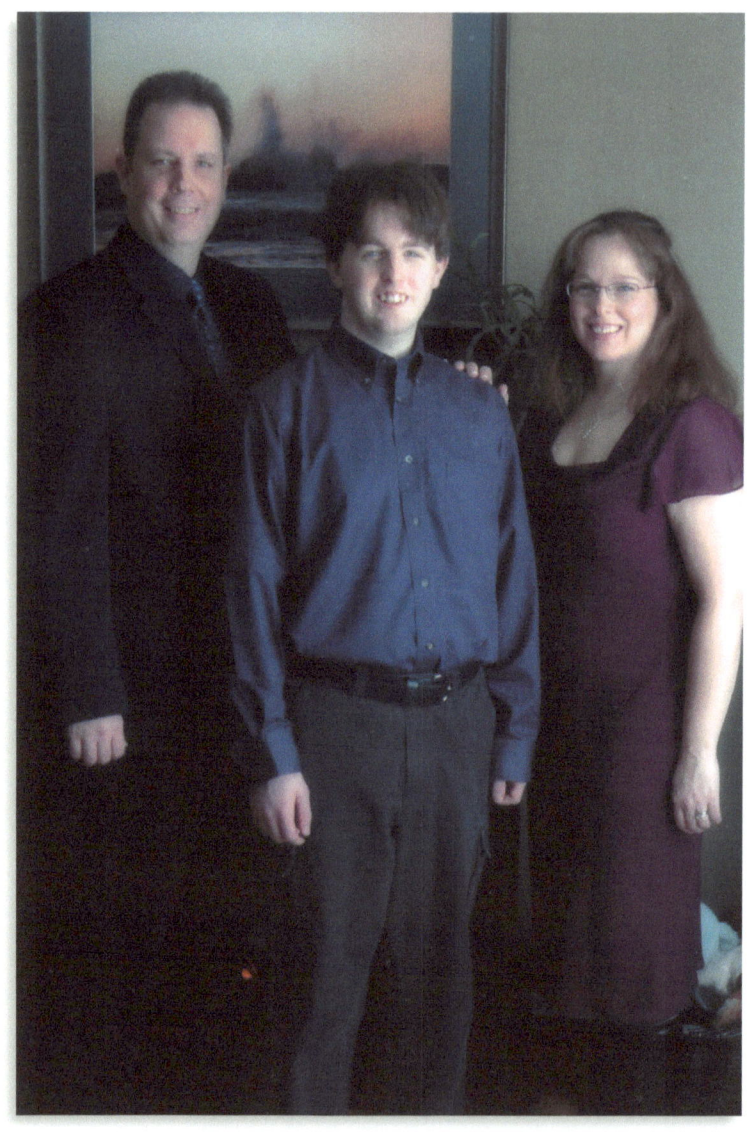

The Nightingale Family. February 18, 2005.
Photo by Jeff Chase.

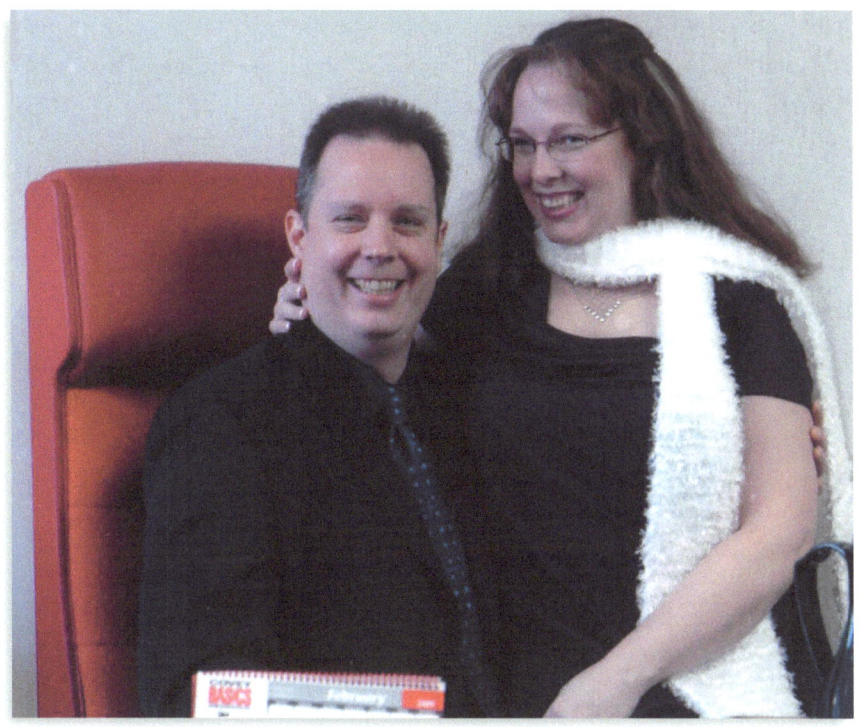

Gary and I goofing off in the judge's chair after we tied the knot. February 18, 2005. Photo by Jeff Chase.

It was an extraordinary day, and everything went as planned. Despite the short notice, many of our friends and family members were able to attend. Our reception started off with a light lunch, cutting the cake, and opening presents, but eventually it turned into an evening party filled with music, drinks, and laughter. Gary and I were thankful we had decided to celebrate our wedding with everyone as we both had a wonderful time. I was grateful to be alive and healthy enough to experience such an amazing, heartwarming event.

Even though it had been fifteen years since my mother had passed away, I still missed her presence every day, especially on my wedding day. My mother was a caring and compassionate lady who never missed an opportunity to tell me how special I was. She encouraged me to explore all of my hopes and dreams, and she made me feel like all things were possible through hard work. I loved my mother dearly. It was a privilege to be her daughter and I was grateful for the time we had together. I wish she could've met Gary; she would've loved him and would've been happy I married such an incredible man.

The following is the journal entry I wrote two days later on the 15th anniversary of my mother's death.

> *Sunday, February 20, 2005: I understand my mother much more now, and I think the more I understand her, the more I forgive her. My mother had a pretty tough life and a very poor marriage so she made different decisions than I would have made. I believe that she did the best she could considering her situation. Not a day goes by that I don't miss my mom in some little way. She was my best friend, and she was often so sad and fragile that I wanted to protect her from the world. I wish I was with her more during the last few months of her life.*

A few weeks later, the results of my blood test came back and everything was normal. I wish I could say this was the end of my issues, but things were about to get much worse.

CHAPTER 17

NEW EYE COMPLICATIONS

Just six weeks after my eye was removed, I started having issues. My ophthalmologist, Dr. Purdy, noticed pustules forming under my eyelid, causing irritation and discharge. He originally thought I was allergic to the acrylic conformer used to shape my new eye after my surgery and thought the issue would clear up once I had my prosthetic eye. Unfortunately, that wasn't the case as the issues continued long after I was fitted with my prosthetic eye.

During 2005 and 2006, I constantly had discharge, irritation, and pain. I also started having chronic headaches and frequent migraines, making my life, at times, unbearable. I went to countless ophthalmologist appointments, often multiple times each month. I was prescribed a variety of drops and medications, but the issues continued. My ophthalmologist thought I might be allergic to the material used to make my prosthetic eye and recommended I find out if my ocularist offered an alternative type of eye. I contacted my ocularist, and I was told they only made acrylic prosthetic eyes.

By November of 2006, I was at my wits' end; I was frustrated and disappointed. Gary and I flew to Toronto to discuss my situation with my surgeon, Dr. McGowan. It was an ominous feeling to be walking through the halls of the Princess Margaret Hospital again, but I was hopeful Dr. McGowan, with his vast knowledge and experience, would be able to help me. He examined me and prescribed two types of eye drops (fluorometholone 0.1% and polyethylene/propylene). He also recommended I see Daphne, a Toronto ocularist, to modify my prosthetic eye so it would not rub against my orbital implant.

Daphne Archibald turned out to be a kind, gentle, soft spoken lady with a bright, beautiful smile. She carefully removed my prosthetic eye and took it away to make some modifications. When she returned, she fit my eye back in place and handed me a mirror. As I looked at myself in the mirror, I had to fight back tears. At that moment I felt like I had my original eye back; I looked like myself again. Gary and I were both in awe of her work as we couldn't see a difference between my prosthetic eye and my real eye. We expressed our gratitude to Daphne and told her we would definitely come back to see her again. With the modifications to my prosthetic eye and the prescribed eye drops, I felt much better. Unfortunately, a few months later, the issues returned.

By the fall of 2007, my eye was feeling especially irritated and painful. One day, I removed my prosthetic with the hope that cleaning it would relieve some of the irritation. I examined my orbital implant and noticed a small, plastic thread sticking out of the centre of it. I immediately wondered if the plastic thread was causing my issues. I met with a local ophthalmologist who recommended I return to Toronto to see my surgeon.

Since Gary was exceptionally busy with work and I was not comfortable going to a large city alone, I asked my best friend, Sherri Chenard, to accompany me. By this point, Sherri and I had known each other for nearly twenty-five years. We met while we were in high school and immediately became close friends. I was drawn to her positivity and excitement for life. Over the years, we supported each other through a variety of life's ups and downs. We always had something to laugh or cry about and could easy talk for hours at any given time. I knew she would be the perfect travelling companion.

Sherri and I flew to Toronto and immediately went to the Princess Margaret Hospital to see Dr. McGowan. He said the donor sclera tissue covering my orbital implant had a stitch exposed. He said it happened occasionally, but it wasn't anything to be concerned about and it should correct itself over time. Dr. McGowan carefully snipped the stitch and sent me on my way. He also recommended I see Daphne again to ensure my prosthetic eye was still fitting properly and not rubbing against my implant. Since Daphne wasn't available, I had my prosthetic eye adjusted by her colleague, Matt. His adjustments made my eye look and feel much better. Afterwards, Sherri and I had a delicious lunch at an authentic Indian restaurant then spent a few hours shopping before catching our flight home. It was a quick trip, but it was productive, and we had fun. I was grateful I had such a wonderful friend who would drop everything and accompany me on such an important trip.

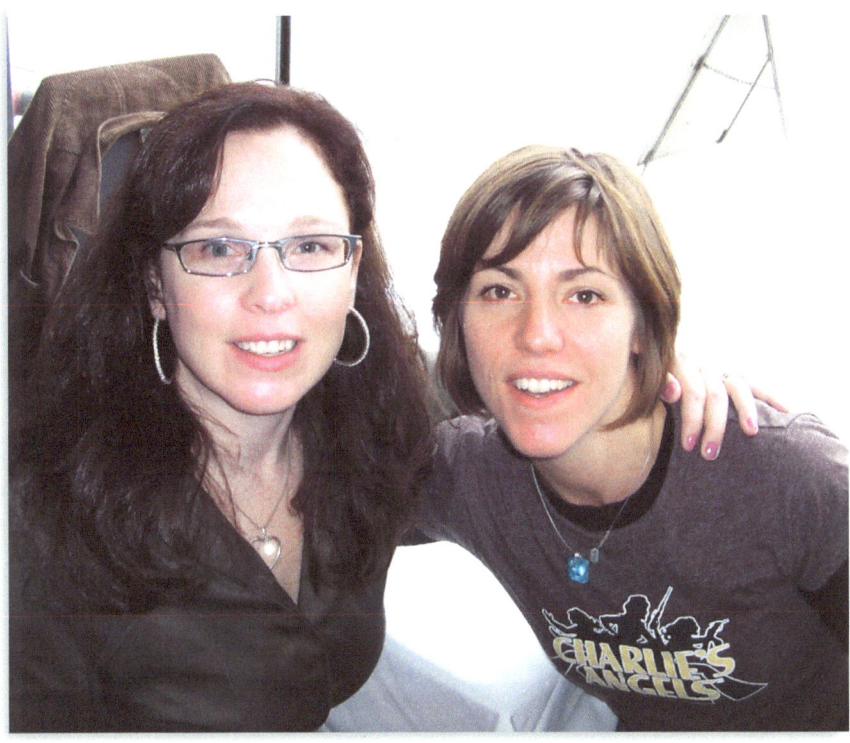

Sherri and I during our Toronto trip while having lunch at a fabulous Indian restaurant.

As much as I wished that was the end of it, less than a year later, another stitch started to reveal itself. That wasn't my only issue though; one morning I woke up to see a spot of blood on my pillowcase. I immediately went to the mirror. As I removed my prosthetic eye, a tear of blood streamed down my face. I looked closely at my implant in the mirror. To my surprise the tissue covering my orbital implant had separated, and I could see the surface of the white ball. I was horrified; I had no idea if or how it could be repaired. After my last experience, I was nervous and depressed at the thought of another surgery and the painful recovery period.

In August 2008, I wrote the following poem about living with chronic pain.

> *Pain.*
> *It can be company, it can be stressful.*
> *It can be tiring and depressing.*
> *It can limit you and it can frighten you.*
> *It can make you angry or feel sad.*
> *It can ruin your day and give you a sleepless night.*
> *It can overpower you and it can disturb you.*
> *Pain does not care about you or your feelings.*

In September 2008, Gary and I flew back to Toronto to see Dr. McGowan yet again. He examined me and immediately referred me to an oculoplastic surgeon who we met later that day. The surgeon said there was an excellent oculoplastic surgeon, Dr. Alejandra Valenzuela, working much closer to our area at the Queen Elizabeth II Hospital (QEII) in Halifax, Nova Scotia. I was grateful to have an option closer to home, but because of the shortage of specialists in our area, I was concerned it would take several months before she could fit me into her schedule. A couple of weeks later, I was relieved when I received a call from Dr. Valenzuela's receptionist with an available appointment.

CHAPTER 18

DARK DAYS

On October 7, 2008, Gary and I drove to Halifax to meet with Dr. Valenzuela. Since Halifax was just a four-hour drive from our home, it was a much more manageable distance than Toronto. Dr. Valenzuela was a tall, young woman. She was very kind and immediately made me feel comfortable.

She examined me and said she would need to sew a patch onto my orbital implant to repair the hole. As I suspected, she said it would take some time before she could fit me into her schedule as she had a backlog of patients. I was disappointed she couldn't fix my implant right away, but I was grateful I found someone willing to help me. I tried my best to remain hopeful.

As the weeks and months passed, I became more defeated and more depressed. I called Dr. Valenzuela's receptionist repeatedly for a surgery date, but she kept telling me there was a long list of people ahead of me with life threatening illnesses, and she didn't know when the doctor would be able to fit me into her schedule. I didn't know what to do. I needed surgery to repair my eye, but I was at the mercy of the system. Pain, headaches, migraines, discharge, and bleeding continued to darken every part of my life. I tried to remain positive, but I wasn't even sure my issues would go away after the doctor repaired my implant.

By March of 2009, I was in constant pain and severely depressed. I was missing a lot of time from work, and barely a day went by without at least one tearful episode. I was feeling anxious at the smallest issue, and I was having heart palpitations and panic attacks.

After my mother died, I went through a very similar dark period. I missed her terribly and I was feeling abandoned and alone. I was working two part-time jobs and attending university while caring for my young son. It was tough to make ends meet. At times, I was worried we would run out of food or have our power disconnected. After a few challenging years, I met Gary and things started to change. He made me laugh and feel loved and he immediately adored little Matt, who looked at him like a superhero. Gary's family embraced us and started inviting Matt and I to all of their family gatherings. Before long, I graduated from university and started working full time. It was a challenging time in my life, but I managed to live through it, and I knew I could live through this too, but I was struggling.

The following is the journal entry I wrote after calling Dr. Valenzuela's office.

> *Monday, March 30, 2009: I am deeply saddened by my life. The doctor has put me off yet again, and it looks like it will be at least July before they can even consider booking my surgery. They said the cancer patients get priority. Well, there will always be cancer patients so I guess they will always get priority. Maybe my eye will never be fixed, maybe I'll live with the pain, bleeding, and discharge forever. I'm so tired. I'm tired of thinking positive and having trust in the system. Where did I go wrong? So many wrong turns took me here. What do I do now? I've lost all my faith in humanity. My life has been consumed by these issues. My joy is gone. I don't know what to live for anymore. I feel so completely out of control. How can I be happy with chronic pain and an open sore for an eye? My entire life has been taken over by my*

> *illness ... I feel like I'm taking everyone down around me. ...*
> *I just feel like a burden.*

Gary was extremely disappointed with the situation as well. He asked me to book another appointment with Dr. Valenzuela right away, and if she couldn't give me a surgery date, we would find another doctor, even if it meant going back to Toronto.

On April 8, 2009, Gary and I drove to Halifax again and met with Dr. Valenzuela. I did my best to impress upon her how badly I was feeling. I told her my implant was constantly bleeding, I had chronic pain, regular migraines, and I was becoming extremely depressed. She examined me again and, to my surprise, she said my orbital implant was so damaged it could no longer be repaired and would need to be removed. The large hole in the sclera tissue had allowed bacteria to get into my porous implant, making it impossible for a patch to heal. Because of my chronic issues, she recommended having a dermis fat graph implant this time. She would harvest some fat and tissue from my abdomen and use it to fill my eye cavity, eliminating the need for donor sclera tissue or an orbital sphere. Like my original implant, the fat graph would be attached to some of my optic muscles, enabling it to have some movement. Since she would only be using my own tissue, I would no longer have an orbital sphere for my body to reject. She reassured me that I shouldn't have any further issues, but she couldn't be 100% sure. She agreed my situation had become much worse and, to my great relief, booked my surgery for June 8, 2009—nearly five years after my first operation. I was worried about the painful recovery period and hoped it wouldn't be as difficult as my first surgery but, at that point, I was willing to go through whatever trauma necessary to fix my issues.

CHAPTER 19

STARTING OVER

On June 6, 2009, Gary and I drove to Halifax. We arrived late, picked up some takeout, and checked into a hotel. The next morning, we went to the QEII Hospital for my pre-surgery assessment and tests. I talked to the anesthesiologist about my extreme nausea and vomiting after my first surgery. He assured me he would give me something during my surgery to prevent a reoccurrence. Afterwards, I had a cardiogram and a blood test. I handled the blood test much better than I did before my first surgery. Over the past five years I had been having blood tests every six months for cancer screening, and I had been working through my fear of needles.

With the rest of the day free, Gary and I went shopping for a few hours and then went out for a nice dinner at a little Italian restaurant. We were both nervous about my surgery and the recovery period, but we were hopeful things were about to change for the better.

The next morning, we got up early and made our way to the hospital. Instead of feeling nervous and sad like I was before my first surgery, I was optimistic and happy I was finally getting rid of my broken implant. I was certain things would get better once it was gone. I checked in, got changed, and waited with Gary until they called my name. They took me into an operating room, put in an IV, and the next thing I knew I was waking up in the recovery room.

When I woke up, I felt some pressure from the tight bandage, otherwise I felt great. Before long, an orderly came to take me back to my hospital room. As I was wheeled through the halls of the hospital, I realized I didn't have a headache for the first time in years. Once I was alone in my room, I crawled around the bars on my bed and walked into the washroom with my IV pole in tow. At that point, Gary came into my room expecting to see me in bad shape, but to his surprise, he found an empty bed. He asked the nurse if she had given him the wrong room number since I was not in my bed. The nurse and Gary rushed back into the room just as I was coming out of the washroom. The two of them scolded me, telling me I shouldn't be out of bed since I had just gotten out of surgery. I laughed and said they should be happy I was feeling so well.

I had a minimal amount of pain and only took acetaminophen as needed. I didn't have any nausea or vomiting, which was a wonderful change from my first surgery. I was back in my room for a few hours before I remembered that Dr. Valenzuela had taken fat and tissue from my abdomen to create my new implant. I pulled up my hospital gown and looked at my stomach. I could see a wide bandage on the lower left side of my stomach, but I didn't feel any pain. Dr. Valenzuela later told me she had made the incision in the same location as my caesarean section scar, knowing I would not likely have any feeling in the scar tissue. Gary stayed by my side for the rest of the day, ducking out occasionally for coffee and treats. To help me recover and avoid blood clots, every couple of hours Gary would hold my hand and lead me through the halls of the hospital for some exercise. Eventually, I sent him back to the hotel to get some much-needed rest. I watched TV for a while and, for the first time in years, I slept through the night.

The next morning, Dr. Valenzuela came in and took off my bandage. She told me everything went as expected and I was healing well. She discharged me and gave me an appointment to have my abdominal stitches removed.

After the doctor left, I got dressed, packed my things, and we headed toward home.

Over the next week, I had some bruising, swelling, pressure, and dizziness, but nothing in comparison to my original surgery. I still made sure to use an ice pack multiple times each day so I could heal as quickly as possible.

Two weeks after my surgery, on a bright sunny day in the middle of June, Gary and I drove back to Halifax for a check-up and to have my abdominal stitches removed. I was feeling good with very little swelling or pain. Dr. Valenzuela said my implant was healing well, and then she painlessly removed the stitches from my abdomen. I told her how much better I was feeling and how grateful I was to her for removing my broken implant. We left the hospital and went to an eclectic pub-style restaurant on Quinpool Road called Freeman's Little New York. We had a delicious meal, a few laughs with our fabulous server, and then headed for home. We enjoyed the drive, discussing our future plans and listening to our favourite music.

CHAPTER 20

WALKING IN HER FOOTSTEPS

A month after my surgery, I was feeling better than I had in years. The pain, headaches, and migraines were gone, and my anxiety and depression had lifted. I was happily getting back to my old routine and finally starting to feel like I did before cancer hijacked my life. I was eating healthy, I started jogging, and I returned to work ahead of schedule.

Since my orbital implant had been removed and was replaced with a dermis fat graph, I wouldn't be able to use my current prosthetic eye because it wouldn't fit properly. I decided to contact Daphne Archibald, the Toronto ocularist, to make my new eye. I was extremely impressed by the adjustments she made to my first prosthetic eye and even though it would mean another trip to Toronto, it would be well worth it.

When I called Daphne to make an appointment, she told me she was planning a trip to PEI in August and she would be able to make my prosthetic eye while she was there. Since PEI was just a three-hour drive away, Gary and I were grateful for the option. Daphne sent me an email with her PEI address, and I was pleasantly surprised—it was just a few kilometres away from my mother's final resting place. It was an amazing coincidence, but it was the perfect ending to my tumultuous journey.

On August 18, 2009, on a beautiful sunny day, Gary and I drove to Hunter River, PEI. Seeing the familiar red soil and the countless fields of patchwork farmland made me feel nostalgic for my childhood summer vacations.

Before my family moved to the Maritimes, each summer we would take a road trip from our home in Ontario to PEI. I fondly remembered singing along to songs on the radio and staying at various motels along the way. On the island, we would stay at a beautiful campground, sleep in a tent-trailer every night and swim in the ocean every day while trying to avoid seaweed and jellyfish. We reconnected with family and friends, had meals cooked on a Coleman stove or a barbeque, and evenings were spent toasting marshmallows around a campfire. As a child, I saw PEI as a magical place, not because of its beauty but because of how happy it made my parents. While we were on the island, their frown lines would disappear, they rarely argued or yelled, and they often smiled and laughed while spending time with friends and family.

Gary and I found the white century home where Daphne was staying and drove up the gravel driveway. We were welcomed by a tall, purple lilac bush swaying in the wind. I was immediately reminded of my mother as she loved the sweet scent of lilacs and, as a child, I often picked them for her. The house felt familiar, as if I was walking into my maternal grandparents' original house near Tignish, PEI. It was a two-story farmhouse with a large kitchen, tall, narrow sash windows, and natural woodwork. We took a seat at the kitchen table, and Daphne started the process of creating my new prosthetic eye. After making a mould and painting an iris, my prosthetic eye needed to cure for a few hours. With Daphne's permission, I cut a bunch of lilac flowers, and Gary and I left to visit my mother's grave.

Before she died, my mother picked out a plot in Floral Hills Memorial Gardens in Hunter River, PEI. She told me she loved the design as it did not have any gravestones or monuments, but instead it had ground plaques and looked more like a nature park than a graveyard. My mother wanted her visitors to have a pleasant experience, enjoy the gardens, and the beautiful scenic views.

We drove into the cemetery, parked, and got out of the car. I immediately felt the strong island wind gusting across the grounds. The air was cool and fresh, a welcome change from the humidity back home. Looking around, I admired the manicured green lawns and raised flowerbeds full of pink and red flowers. There were also rows of green hedges, multiple flowering bushes, and mature trees strategically placed throughout to provide shade. As we walked up to my mother's plot, I couldn't help noticing how separated it was from most of the others, and it seemed lonely. I felt sad to see her name written on her plaque; it made me miss her a little more. I thought about all of our missed opportunities to experience life together. I longed to hug my mother and protect her from the harshness of the world. I wiped away a few stray clippings of freshly cut grass from her plaque and placed the bouquet of lilacs on her grave. Gary held me as I shed a few tears for my mother and the void her death left in my life. Having just gone through my own battle with cancer, I felt closer to her than ever. Gary and I strolled hand in hand around the grounds in the bright sunshine; before long a feeling of calmness came over me. I was comforted knowing I was walking on the same red dirt roads my mother had walked on many years before.

Later that afternoon, we returned to Daphne's where I was fitted with my new prosthetic eye. As usual, Daphne made it look and feel amazing. We said our goodbyes and headed toward home feeling confident our journey had come to an end.

In the months and years that followed, Dr. Valenzuela would be proven right as my issues would be almost completely eliminated by using a dermis fat graph implant. Occasionally, I would still get headaches from too much eye strain, but the chronic pain was gone, and my quality of life greatly improved. The phantom eye syndrome with the lights and shadows never went away but, as Dr. Purdy had predicted, eventually I got used to it. It took several years but, with some effort, I learned to adjust to my missing depth perception and the changes in my vision so I could once again appreciate the beauty of nature.

This experience made me extremely grateful for the love and support of my family, friends, and especially my wonderful husband and son. During this period, I learned a great deal about myself and my shortcomings. I realized being out of control made me frustrated and angry. I had to learn that some things are completely beyond my control, however, at the same time, I had to keep in mind that a great number of things, including my attitude, are within my control so I should not feel helpless. I realized how important it was to be flexible in my expectations so I wouldn't become completely devastated and disappointed when things turned out differently than I expected. Finally, I also realized that I am not just my body or my outward appearance; I am a complex, deeply sensitive person with a desire to help others in my own unique way.

I wish I could say this was the end of my health issues, but I would have many more trials and tribulations to come. The strength and purpose I found from this experience would help me face my future issues with grace and positivity.

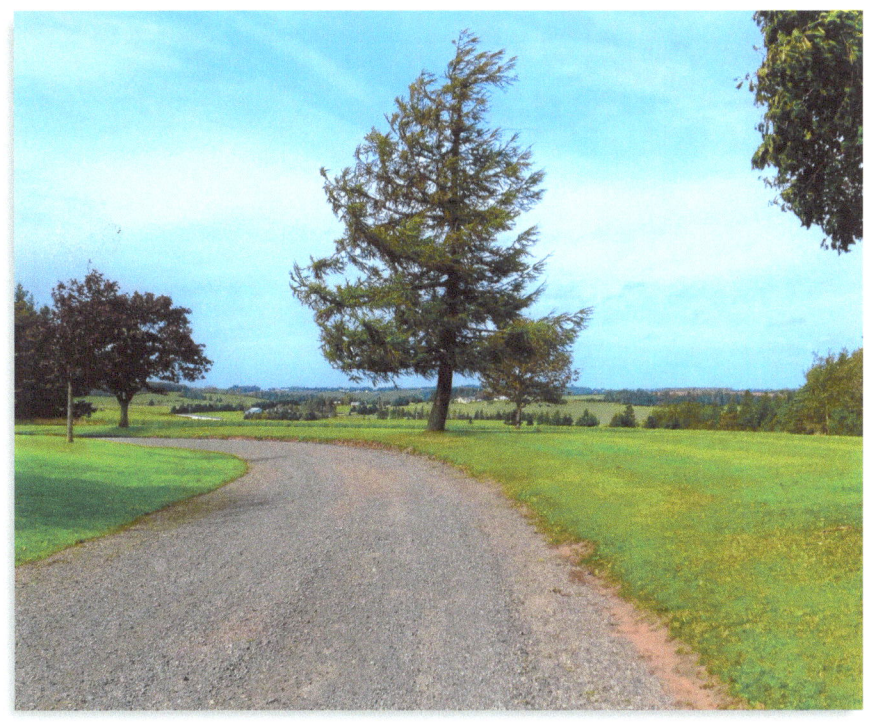

My mother's final resting place in Floral Hills Memorial Gardens in beautiful Prince Edward Island.

Thank you for reading my story.
I hope it can be of some help.
C

CPSIA information can be obtained
at www.ICGtesting.com
Printed in the USA
LVHW070000030221
678156LV00007B/10